All about Your Eyes

All about Your Eyes

SECOND EDITION, REVISED AND UPDATED

EDITED BY SHARON FEKRAT, MD, FACS,

HENRY FENG, MD, AND TANYA S. GLASER, MD

DUKE UNIVERSITY PRESS DURHAM & LONDON 2021

Project editor: Jessica Ryan
Designed by Amy Ruth Buchanan
Typeset in Minion Pro by Copperline Book Services.

Library of Congress Cataloging-in-Publication Data
Names: Fekrat, Sharon, editor. | Glaser, Tanya S., [date] editor. |
Feng, Henry L., [date] editor.
Title: All about your eyes / edited by Sharon Fekrat, MD, FACS,
Henry Feng, MD, Tanya S. Glaser, MD
Description: Second edition, revised and updated. | Durham :
Duke University Press, 2021. | Includes index.
Identifiers: LCCN 2020038093 (print)
LCCN 2020038094 (ebook)
ISBN 9781478010500 (hardcover)
ISBN 9781478011606 (paperback)
ISBN 9781478021209 (ebook)
Subjects: LCSH: Eye—Diseases. | Ophthalmology.
Classification: LCC RE46 .A44 2021 (print) | LCC RE46 (ebook) |
DDC617.7/1—dc23
LC record available at https://lccn.loc.gov/2020038093
LC ebook record available at https://lccn.loc.gov/2020038094

Cover art © Ashley Slocum

Contents

12 • Infection and Inflammation of the Eye

13 • Tumors of the Eye and Orbit

14 • The Optic Nerve

Illustrations

Foreword

EDWARD BUCKLEY, MD

In today's rapidly changing healthcare environment, patients are being met with more challenges and choices than ever before when it comes to navigating their medical care. Ranging from a variety of insurance plans to complex treatment regimens, it is not surprising to learn that older patients often have the most difficulty understanding and utilizing the full range of healthcare services.

This is particularly important in terms of eye disease as the likelihood of developing visual impairment increases with age. Leading causes of decreased vision include cataract, glaucoma, macular degeneration, and diabetic retinopathy, all of which are more common and often more severe in older individuals. Fortunately, novel therapies continue to be developed for many of these sight-threatening conditions, allowing vision to be preserved for many more people. However, as the population grows, physicians are also met with increasing demands for care, resulting in pressures to see more patients and a reduction in the amount of available time for patient education and counseling.

Healthcare leaders continue to recognize the importance of patient-centered, integrative, and personalized medicine as an integral part of a successful healthcare experience. As such, patients are often met with various diagnostic and treatment decisions, many of which may be difficult to fully understand. Even with the burgeoning wealth of information on the Internet, it may be difficult for many to understand medical topics described on certain websites, and even more challenging to ensure that those sources are reputable and updated. Nonetheless, many of today's patients are excellent advocates for their own health and often demand detailed information when possible.

In order to meet the continually growing need for patient education, Drs. Sharon Fekrat, Henry Feng, and Tanya Glaser have organized and updated an important, detailed, yet readable handbook designed to help those who are interested in eye health better understand certain eye conditions and participate in their own eye care. This second edition extends critical knowledge about eye disease from some of our country's best eye doctors to interested readers, and ultimately impacts not just patients, but also their family and friends.

The early chapters discuss basic eye anatomy, function, and refractive correction. The book then goes on to highlight some of the most important eye conditions as identified by the National Eye Institute and the World Health Organization. In most instances, the text is organized by specific disease, but it also expands upon novel medications, imaging tests, and surgical procedures to help demystify the most impactful eye conditions and available treatments.

All about Your Eyes is a remarkably detailed yet understandable resource that will surely empower patients and their family members with the knowledge needed to participate in their own eye care.

Introduction

SHARON FEKRAT, MD, FACS, HENRY FENG, MD,
AND TANYA S. GLASER, MD

It has been almost 15 years since the first edition of *All about Your Eyes* was published in 2006. Since that time, there have been many advances in the diagnosis and treatment of eye disease. To keep the readership up-to-date with the latest information, we thought that it was time for a second edition.

We have maintained the same general format but have added new sections on cutting-edge imaging modalities such as fundus autofluoresence and OCT angiography, and updated sections to include the latest treatment options, such as femtosecond laser during cataract surgery and retinal prostheses, just to name a few.

On behalf of all the eye doctors who have trained at or are currently working at the Duke Eye Center, we hope that you and your family and friends benefit from the information contained herein. Although reading about your eyes in this book can provide a useful understanding of the eyes and the various conditions that may affect them, this book is not designed to promote self-diagnosis or be a substitute for a visit to your eye doctor. Only after a thorough eye examination and any necessary testing can your eye doctor come up with an accurate diagnosis and treatment plan.

1 · Anatomy of the Eye and How It Works

Eyelids

JAMES H. POWERS, MD

The eyelids serve two principal functions: protection and lubrication of the eye. The eyelids protect the eye by acting as a physical barrier that prevents both excessive light and foreign objects from damaging the eye, while eyelashes trap unwanted debris. The eyelid lubricates the eye by distributing the tear film evenly across the surface of the eye. Tiny glands in the eyelid add oil to the tear film to help prevent evaporation.

Anatomically, the eyelid is composed of an outer layer of skin, followed by a layer of muscle and supportive tissue, and finally the innermost conjunctiva. The muscular layer helps control the opening and closing of the eyelid. The conjunctiva of the eyelid is continuous with that of the eyeball. The eyelid can be affected by both acquired and congenital disorders, including infection, inflammation, neurologic disorders, anatomic abnormalities, and malignancy.

Conjunctiva

TANYA GLASER, MD

The conjunctiva is a thin mucous membrane that covers the white (sclera) of the eye and the inner surface of the upper and lower eyelids. The conjunctiva becomes thinner as it nears the cornea (the clear front circular surface of the eye) and terminates at the edge (limbus) of the cornea. The conjunctiva serves as the outer protective covering of the eyeball and provides a smooth surface that interfaces with the eyelids, making blinking and eye movements comfortable. Blood vessels in the conjunctiva help nourish the eye. Blood or inflammation in the conjunctiva, such as with subconjunctival hemorrhage or conjunctivitis, can cause it to appear red or pink.

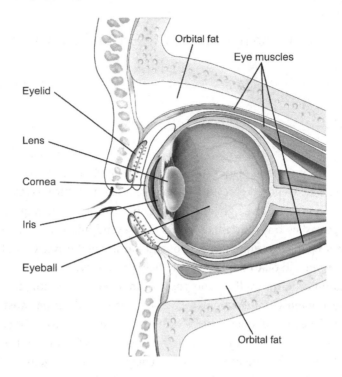

Orbital fat

Eye muscles

Eyelid

Lens

Cornea

Iris

Eyeball

Orbital fat

1.1. Side view of the eyeball behind the eyelids.

Sclera

NIKOLAS RAUFI, MD

The sclera is the outer tough, white connective tissue that forms the eye wall. It begins at the edge of the clear cornea, called the limbus, and extends backward toward the optic nerve. The "white part" of the eye is actually the sclera covered by a thin layer of tissue called conjunctiva. The sclera is made of collagen fibers, which provide strength and support, giving structure to the eyeball. In the back of the eye, the sclera provides attachments for the darkly pigmented choroid on its inner surface. It also serves as the attachment site for the six eye muscles. Contraction of these eye muscles pulls on the sclera and causes the eye to move. Like other parts of the eye, problems can occur in the sclera; scleritis and episcleritis are two examples of inflammatory scleral conditions.

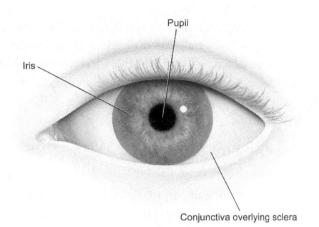

1.2. Front view of the eyeball.

Cornea

C. ELLIS WISELY, MD, MBA

The cornea is the transparent, round, dome-shaped tissue on the front central surface of the eye and is the window through which light passes into the eye. A normal cornea has a diameter of 12 millimeters (mm) and a thickness of 0.5 mm. The cornea is made up of thin layers of proteins and cells stacked upon one another. The cornea's innermost layer, called the corneal endothelium, acts as a pump to remove water from the cornea, allowing the cornea to remain clear.

Unlike other parts of the eye, the cornea does not have a blood supply. Thus, to get oxygen and nutrients, the cornea absorbs substances circulating in the tears and in the aqueous humor (fluid inside the front part of the eye). The cornea is one of the most densely innervated tissues in the body, making it painful to touch or scratch.

Protecting the eye and focusing the light that enters the eye are two principal functions of the cornea. The cornea protects the eye by providing a physical barrier against pathogens such as bacteria, by harboring immune cells, and by sending pain signals in the event of injury. The dome-shaped curve of the cornea allows it to bend and focus light, a process called refraction, on the center of the retina so we can see clearly. The cornea actually provides more refractive power than the lens of the eye. Alterations in the normal, curved shape of the cornea can result in astigmatism, nearsightedness, and farsightedness. Disruption of the tear film can lead to dry eye, which can affect the cornea's refracting ability and cause blurry vision.

Iris and Ciliary Body

JENNIFER LIRA, MD

The iris is the round, colored part of the eye with a smaller, dark, round opening in its center called the pupil. The iris can range in color from blue to green to brown, depending on how much pigment (melanin) it contains and how thick the iris tissue is. A brown iris has more melanin-containing cells than a blue iris. The color of the iris also affects how long dilation eye drops last, with lighter-colored irises typically having longer dilation periods. Eye doctors use dilating eye drops to pharmacologically enlarge the pupil in order to see through it and examine all the eye structures behind the iris. The iris adjusts to allow the pupil to get smaller in brighter lighting and larger in dimmer lighting.

The iris structurally divides the front part of the eye into two compartments, the anterior and posterior chambers. The anterior chamber is in front of the iris and the posterior chamber is behind the iris. Just behind the outer edge of the iris is the ciliary body, a structure that makes aqueous humor (the clear fluid inside the front of the eye) and also serves as an attachment point for the zonules. Zonules are thin fibers that support and suspend the lens inside the eye. The muscles of the ciliary body contract and relax to control the lens shape, thereby allowing the eye to focus on near or distant objects.

Pupil

JENNIFER LIRA, MD

The pupil is the opening in the center of the iris (the colored part of the eye). Light passes through the pupil and lens to reach the retina, which then sends signals to the brain to form an image. The size of the pupil controls the amount of light entering the eye. The pupil becomes smaller in bright light conditions, which reduces peripheral blur and increases depth of focus. The pupil also becomes smaller when focusing at near, a process called accommodation. In contrast, the pupil becomes larger in dark conditions in order to allow as much light in as possible to maximize vision.

The iris controls the size of the pupil through two sets of muscles. One muscle is oriented radially like the spokes on a bicycle wheel and dilates the pupil. The other muscle is ring-shaped and encircles the pupil to constrict it. Both the visual system and the body's central nervous system control these muscles to let in the appropriate amount of light.

The average diameter of the pupil is approximately 3–4 mm in ambient light conditions. Because the size of the pupil is regulated by the visual system, which includes both the eye and the brain, checking the pupillary reaction to light is a basic test of brain function. Eye doctors also check the pupillary response to light in order to evaluate how the eyes perceive light in comparison to each other.

Chambers

RAVI CHANDRASHEKHAR, MD, MSEE

The space inside the front part of the eyeball is divided into two main areas, or chambers. The front or anterior chamber is the space between the cornea and the front of the iris. The back or posterior chamber is between the back of the iris and the front of the vitreous gel. These chambers are filled with aqueous humor, a clear fluid produced by the eye to nourish itself. The aqueous humor normally drains out through the anterior chamber angle, which is at the edges of where the cornea meets the iris. This balance between production and drainage of aqueous humor helps to maintain a healthy eye pressure.

Lens

MARK GOERLITZ-JESSEN, MD

The lens of the eye is located in the posterior chamber, behind the iris and pupil and directly in front of the vitreous gel. The lens is made of transparent proteins, called crystallins, that allow light to pass from the front to the back of the eye. As light passes through the lens it is bent and focused, a process known as refraction, onto the retina in the back of the eye. The lens contributes approximately 30% of the focusing power of the eye, while the remaining 70% comes from the cornea.

The lens resides inside a thin capsule, or "bag," which is suspended in place by zonules. These zonules are connected to a circular muscle on the eye wall called the ciliary body. When a person looks at something up close, the ciliary body and zonules alter the shape of the lens to allow the eye to maintain focus. The change in lens shape for focusing at near is called accommodation. As we age, the lens thickens and becomes stiff, decreasing its ability to change shape and as a result, near vision becomes out of focus. This is why with age, we begin to need reading glasses.

Over time, the lens becomes larger, denser, and cloudy, giving it a yellow-brown appearance. These changes to the lens are what is known as a cataract. Cataract formation is a normal part of aging but can lead to decreased vision. The treatment for cataracts is cataract surgery and implantation of a synthetic intraocular lens.

Vitreous

FAITH A. BIRNBAUM, MD

The vitreous is a clear gel-like material that fills the eyeball behind the iris-lens diaphragm and extends back to the retina to which it is attached at birth. The vitreous gel is denser and firmer in youth and becomes more liquid with age. In normal aging, the back of the vitreous gel can pull away from the retina, known as a posterior vitreous detachment, which can result in floaters. Occasionally, separation of the vitreous gel from the retinal surface can cause retinal breaks in areas where the vitreous and retina were firmly attached.

Retina

JAMES H. POWERS, MD

The retina is a complex layer of nerve tissue located at the back of the eyeball, lining the inner surface of the eye wall. The retina is located between the vitreous (clear gel that fills the back of the eyeball) and the choroid (the blood vessel layer underneath the Bruch membrane). The retina's most peripheral edge is at the ora serrata and the most posterior edge is at the border of the optic nerve. The macula is the most visually important part of the retina and is responsible for detailed central vision. The fovea is an even smaller part of the central macula where visual acuity is sharpest. The retina receives its own blood circulation via the central retinal artery and vein, which brings nutrients and oxygen and removes waste products.

The function of the retina is to convert light into neurochemical signals that are sent to the visual processing centers of the brain, resulting in the perception of vision. The retina accomplishes this complicated task through the action of ten cell layers. Specialized cells called rod photoreceptors process grayscale vision, while cone photoreceptors process color vision. Photoreceptors are critical to vision as they are the first step in the cascade that converts light rays into electrical signals. These electrical signals are then carried to the brain by way of the optic nerve. The macula has a high density of cones and is responsible for detailed colored vision, while the peripheral retina has a higher density of rods and is responsible for night vision.

Retinal Pigment Epithelium and Bruch Membrane

NISHA MUKHERJEE, MD

The retinal pigment epithelium and Bruch membrane are two important tissue layers that line the inside of the eyeball and separate the inner retina from the outer choroid. The retinal pigment epithelium is a single layer of pigment cells that lies directly beneath the retina. These cells are tightly joined to each other and form a barrier between the retina and the choroid. The retinal pigment epithelial cells provide nutrients to the overlying rod and cone photoreceptors in the retina to maintain their proper functioning. When there is loss of the retinal pigment epithelium, there is corresponding loss of the overlying photoreceptors, leading to vision loss. Under the retinal pigment epithelium is the Bruch membrane. The purpose of this tissue layer is to separate the retina and retinal pigment epithelium from the underlying choroid layer. In all eyes, lipids and other materials can build up within the Bruch membrane. In wet age-related macular degeneration, abnormal choroidal blood vessels may grow through breaks in the Bruch membrane and leak fluid or blood underneath the retinal pigment epithelium and/or the retina, resulting in central vision loss.

Choroid

MELISSA MEI-HSIA CHAN, MBBS AND NISHA MUKHERJEE, MD

The choroid is a layer of pigmented vascular tissue that lies between the retina and the sclera (the white connective tissue that makes up the eye wall). It contains many blood vessels that bring in necessary nutrients and oxygen. Since the outer retina has a very high metabolic demand, it needs a large amount of blood flow; this is fulfilled by the choroid, which has the highest blood flow rate of any tissue in the body. The high rate of blood flow in the choroid helps remove thermal energy from the light absorption in the retina. The choroid along with the ciliary body and iris together are known as the uvea. In addition to supplying oxygen and nutrients, the uvea is pigmented with melanin. This pigmentation absorbs excess light entering the eye and limits the amount of light reflected in the eye.

Optic Nerve

KATY C. LIU, MD, PHD

The optic nerve is the "cable" that connects the eye to the brain. Like a fiberoptic cable, the optic nerve comprises a bundle of over one million nerve fibers that carry visual information from the eye to the visual cortex located in the back area of the brain. Each eye has its own optic nerve, which join together behind the eyes at the optic chiasm.

The optic nerve is nourished by blood and oxygen from several blood vessels, including the central retinal artery. The blood supplying the optic nerve returns to the body through the central retinal vein. The optic nerve is protected by several layers of thin, fibrous coverings called meninges that also surround the rest of the brain.

As the cable that connects your eye to your brain, the optic nerve is essential for your vision. The optic nerve can be injured by inflammation, ischemia (lack of blood flow), compression (by the surrounding tissue, a mass, or a tumor), trauma, or elevated eye pressure (also known as glaucoma). Optic nerve injury, in effect, "cuts the cord" and impairs the transmission of visual information to the brain. Damage to the optic nerve can lead to temporary or permanent vision loss.

It is important to assess the health of your optic nerves. Eye doctors such as glaucoma specialists and neuro-ophthalmologists specialize in diseases of the optic nerve. During a dilated eye examination, your eye doctor can examine the front part of the optic nerve that enters the eyeball for signs of damage or disease. The remaining length of the optic nerve cannot be visualized during a routine eye examination, but if there is suspicion for posterior optic nerve damage, your doctor can order brain imaging—a computed tomography (CT) scan or magnetic resonance imaging (MRI) scan—to assess the health of the optic nerves behind the eye.

Orbit

JANE S. KIM, MD

The orbit is the bony socket in the skull in which the eye and all of its appendages, including the extraocular muscles, fascial tissue, fat, nerves, blood vessels, lacrimal gland, lacrimal sac, and nasolacrimal duct, are housed. There are seven bones that make up the four walls of the orbit, providing the structural support needed to protect the eye from direct injury. Most of the orbital volume is composed of orbital fat, which provides cushioning for the eyeball and the extraocular muscles. Within the orbit, there are six extraocular muscles that attach to the sclera and move the eye. The lacrimal gland, lacrimal sac, and nasolacrimal duct are also located within the orbit and function together to lubricate the eye and drain tears. Blood vessels and nerves enter the orbit through several bony openings to provide blood supply and innervation to the eye and all of the structures within the orbit. Finally, the optic nerve passes through an opening at the back of the orbit, called the optic canal, to reach the brain.

Pathways from the Eye to the Brain

OBINNA UMUNAKWE, MD, PHD

The eyes and brain work together to allow you to see and understand your surroundings. The visual pathway begins when light from the outside world enters the eyes. The cornea and lens focus light onto the retina, where special nerve cells called photoreceptors convert the light into electrochemical signals that travel along nerve fibers. Fibers from those nerve cells collectively form the optic nerve, which connects the eye to the brain.

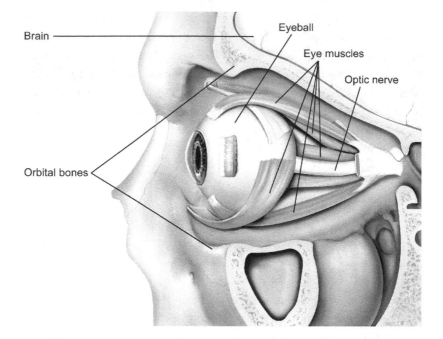

1.3. The eyeball sits in the orbit and has eye muscles attached to it.

One optic nerve from each eye enters the skull through the optic canal at the back of the orbit. After entering the skull, the optic nerves from each eye meet at the optic chiasm. At this point, approximately half of the nerve fibers from the right optic nerve cross over to the left side, and half of the fibers from the left optic nerve cross over to the right side. After the optic chiasm, nerve fibers continue their journey to the brain in the right and left optic tracts. Because of the nerve fibers crossing at the optic chiasm, each optic tract contains nerve fibers from both eyes. Next, each optic tract connects to a portion of the brain called the thalamus. The thalamus sends signals through the white matter of the brain to the visual cortex, located at the back of the brain. In the visual cortex, the brain processes these signals into images.

The perception of vision requires that the entire pathway from the eyes to the visual cortex in the brain be intact. Interruption at any point along the visual pathway leads to loss of vision.

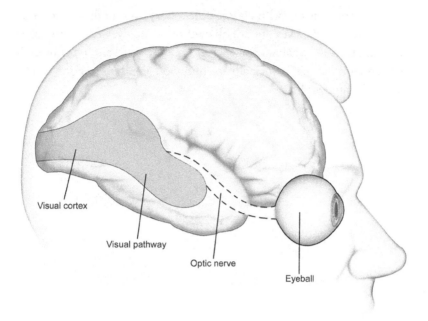

1.4. The visual pathway connects the eyeballs to the brain.

How the Eye Works

OBINNA UMUNAKWE, MD, PHD

The structures in your eye work together to convert light from the environment into images that are interpreted by the brain. The cornea and lens of the eye refract the light to bring images into sharp focus on the retina. The retina converts images into signals that are sent through the optic nerve to the brain for interpretation.

Each eye sends a slightly different image to the brain. You can test this yourself by covering one eye, then the other. The brain combines the images from each eye into a single image, a process known as fusion. This process allows you to have depth perception, which is the ability to see your surroundings in three dimensions (3D). If the vision is decreased or completely lost in one eye, then depth perception is lost.

Fusion is a complicated visual process that develops in childhood. In order for fusion to develop properly, both eyes must have equal visual input and good vision (with glasses if necessary) and both eyes must be in alignment. If the eyes are not aligned or if one eye sees poorly or is occluded, then the images from each eye are too different to be fused. If fusion does not develop normally in childhood, depth perception will be limited throughout life.

Recommended Schedule for Eye Exams

TANYA S. GLASER, MD

Eye examinations are recommended throughout life to ensure the eyes remain healthy and that good vision develops and is maintained. Routine eye exams allow the eye doctor to identify problems that can be corrected in order to prevent vision loss.

Vision screenings are performed on newborn babies by an eye doctor or pediatrician to ensure that there is no obstruction in the visual pathway (such as congenital cataracts), that each eye sees well, and that the eyes are straight and aligned together. Vision screenings should be performed between 6 and 12 months of age, between 3 and 5 years of age, before first grade, and then annually. At the age of 5 or when the child begins school, a formal eye exam is recommended so that the visual acuity, or level of vision, can be measured accurately.

Once vision has developed completely in adults (aged 20 to 39 years), a full comprehensive eye exam, including pharmacologic dilation, every ten years may be sufficient. Adults with known eye problems, risk factors for eye disease (such as diabetes), and those who wear glasses or contact lenses need more frequent exams. Individuals without risk factors for eye disease between the ages of 40 and 64 should undergo a full exam about every 2 years. Around age 65, eye exams are recommended every 1 to 2 years as the incidence of ocular disease increases with age. People with known eye problems may need to be examined more often. Patients with diabetes should be examined at least yearly and sometimes more often, depending on the severity of diabetic eye disease.

Additional Resources

https://www.aao.org/eye-health/tips-prevention-list

https://www.aoa.org/patients-and-public/caring-for-your-vision/comprehensive
    -eye-and-vision-examination/recommended-examination-frequency-for
    -pediatric-patients-and-adults

Eye Care Specialists: Opticians, Optometrists, and Eye MDs (Ophthalmologists), and Ophthalmic Allied Health Professionals

TANYA S. GLASER, MD

Opticians • Opticians are professionals who fit and dispense corrective eyewear including glasses, contact lenses, low vision aids, and ocular prostheses (artificial, non-seeing eyes). Opticians need to complete either a 6-month apprenticeship program or a year-long certificate program, or earn a two-year Associate's Degree in Ophthalmic Dispensing. After this training, opticians can apply to become licensed or certified, depending on the requirements of the state in which they practice.

Optometrists • Optometrists receive a Doctor of Optometry (OD) degree after receiving training in prescribing glasses and contact lenses, rehabilitating the visually impaired, and diagnosing and medically treating certain ocular diseases. Optometrists do not attend medical school. They do not perform surgery and usually do not perform laser treatments. To obtain an OD degree, one must successfully complete a 4-year accredited degree program at a school or college of optometry. Some optometrists complete an optional residency in a specific area of practice. Optometrists must be licensed by the state in which they practice. In several states, optometrists have successfully lobbied to obtain surgical privileges, allowing them to perform selective surgical procedures. Performing surgical procedures remains outside of the scope of practice for optometrists in most states.

Eye MDs (Ophthalmologists) • Ophthalmology is a branch of medicine specializing in the anatomy, function, disease, and medical and surgical treatment of the eye. An ophthalmologist, can provide the full spectrum of eye care, from prescribing glasses and contact lenses to complex medical and surgical treatments for all known eye conditions. Many ophthalmologists are also involved in the scientific research of eye diseases. An ophthalmologist is a medical doctor (that is, an MD, or less commonly, a DO, Doctor of Osteopathic Medicine). After 4 years of medical school and 1 year of medical or surgical internship, every ophthalmologist spends a minimum of 3 years in ophthalmology residency (hospital-based training). Often an ophthalmologist spends an additional 1–2 years training in a subspecialty, or specific area, of eye care (such as glaucoma, medical and/or surgical retina, oculoplastics, neuro-ophthalmology, cornea and refractive ophthalmology, or pediatric ophthalmology). Almost all ophthalmologists are board certified, meaning that they have passed a rigorous written and oral examination given by the American Board of Ophthalmology designed to assess their knowledge, experience, and skills. Technically, anyone with an MD can set up a practice, so make sure that your ophthalmologist is board certified. Like all MDs, ophthalmologists must be licensed in the state in which they practice.

Ophthalmic Allied Health Professionals • Certified Ophthalmic Assistants (COA), Certified Ophthalmic Technicians (COT), and Certified Ophthalmic Medical Technologists (COMT) help comprise the eye care team. These certifications require a study course or training program with increasing requirements from COA (entry level) to COMT (highest level of training). You may interact with COAS, COTS, and COMTs during your visit to your eye doctor as they will often complete your initial assessment, refraction, education, and imaging.

Additional Resources

https://www.aoa.org/about-the-aoa/what-is-a-doctor-of-optometry
https://www.opticianedu.org/optician-vs-optometrist/
https://www.aao.org/eye-health/tips-prevention/what-is-ophthalmologist
https://www.opticiantraining.org/ophthalmic-assistant-technician-technologist
   -certification/

The Eye Exam

TANYA S. GLASER, MD

Eye exams in children and adults have slightly different goals. For children, the most important part of the exam is to ensure the development of normal binocular vision, in which both eyes work together to perceive depth (3D vision). With adults, the goal of the eye exam is to maximize the visual potential and to maintain good vision. Despite these differences, many components of the eye exam remain similar for all ages.

In all cases, the first part of the eye exam is a thorough medical and ocular history. The eye doctor or eye technician may ask you about any vision problems or associated symptoms. For example, do you wear glasses or contact lenses? Have you had any prior eye diseases, eye surgeries, or eye injuries? Reviewing your family history for eye diseases such as glaucoma, diabetes, and age-related macular degeneration can help the eye doctor screen for these conditions early. Also, reviewing any other medical problems and medications helps to assess related health problems.

A comprehensive eye exam then assesses the function and anatomy of each eye. This includes testing the visual acuity, or level of vision, in each eye. Using one eye at a time, you will be asked to read the eye chart, sometimes at more than one distance and often while wearing glasses or contact lenses. A vision of 20/20 means that you see clearly at 20 feet what should normally be seen at that 20 feet. A vision of 20/200 means that you must be as close as 20 feet to see what should normally be seen at 200 feet. If the vision is worse than 20/20, a refraction may be performed to determine what the vision would be if the refractive error were corrected with glasses or contact lenses. Eye alignment and motility (ability to move) are tested to ensure that both eyes are straight and that they move together in all directions. The pupils are checked to make sure that the two pupils are equal in size and respond normally to light. Eye pressure is measured using one of several methods. Each eye's visual field, or peripheral vision, is also checked. The external appearance of the eyes and eyelids are evaluated for proper position and to ensure that the eyes can open and close normally. Sometimes color vision is also measured.

The eye doctor then examines each eye with a slit lamp (a special type of microscope), starting with the front of the eye and moving toward the back of the eye. The eyelids, eyelashes, conjunctiva, sclera, cornea, iris, and anterior chamber are examined for any abnormalities. Then the pupils are usually dilated with eye drops to inspect the eye structures behind the iris. Dilation drops take about 30 minutes to work. After dilation, the pupils can remain dilated and the vision may stay blurry for 4 to 24 hours depending on the type of eye drops used. During a dilated exam, the eye doctor examines the lens, vitreous, retina, and optic nerve head, often using special lenses. If problems are noted during this comprehensive exam, then other tests may be ordered by the eye doctor. For example, computerized visual field testing and optical coherence tomography (OCT) imaging is commonly performed for evaluation of glaucoma and other causes of vision loss. Photographs of the eyes may be taken, and a dye test may be done to determine if there is normal blood flow inside the eyes. Computed tomography (CT) scans and magnetic resonance imaging (MRI) scans of the orbits and brain are performed if problems are suspected in the visual pathways behind the eye that cannot be seen in an eye exam.

Additional Resource

https://www.aao.org/eye-health/tips-prevention/eye-exams-101

3 · Why Do I Need Glasses?

Nearsightedness

MICHELLE SY GO, MS, MD

What Is It? • Nearsightedness, also known as myopia, occurs when the focusing power of the eye is too strong for the length of the eyeball. The image then lands too far in front of the retina within the eye, causing it to be blurry instead of clear. This can happen either because your eye is longer than normal, as in axial myopia, or because the cornea or the lens in the front of the eye has too much focusing power, as in refractive myopia. People with nearsightedness can see better up close than far away.

Nearsightedness most commonly arises during adolescence when the body and eyeball are rapidly changing. It affects over 40% of working-aged adults in the United States. It is very common in East Asia, where 70–85% of adolescents are affected. It is not fully known what causes nearsightedness, but it tends to run in families and is more common in children who were born prematurely. Other risk factors may include prolonged reading and decreased exposure to sunlight during childhood.

Symptoms: What You May Experience • Nearsightedness causes distant objects to be blurry while objects at near are typically clear. You may need to squint or bring objects closer to your face in order to see. Children may have trouble in school because they cannot see the chalkboard or the slides. People who drive may find it difficult to read road signs.

Examination Findings: What the Doctor Looks For • Those with nearsightedness will usually see the visual acuity chart better through pinholes and with lens correction using, for example, glasses or contact lenses. For the majority of people, the rest of the exam is normal. However, those with high myopia, with more than −6 diopters (a unit of refractive power) of correction, may have thinning at the outer edges of the retina called lattice degeneration and are at risk for retinal breaks. In severe cases, such as pathologic myopia, there can be splitting in the ret-

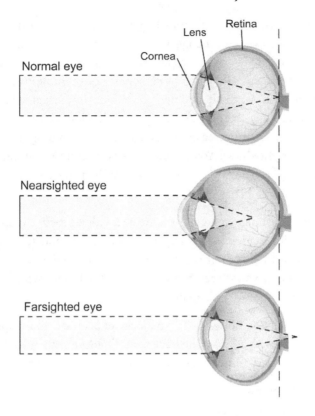

3.1. Top: normal eye. Center: light focuses too far forward in nearsighted eye. Right: light focuses too far back in farsighted eye.

inal layers (retinoschisis), breaks in the macula (lacquer cracks), or the development of abnormal blood vessels (choroidal neovascularization).

What You Can Do • There is ongoing research regarding methods to prevent or slow the progression of nearsightedness, mainly in children in East Asia where myopia is widespread. In these populations, there is evidence that low dose atropine eye drops and exposure to sunlight may slow the incidence or progression rate of rapidly progressing myopia.

When to Call the Doctor • If you are struggling with activities involving distance vision, you should call your eye doctor to schedule a routine eye exam. If you currently wear corrective lenses and your vision is not as clear as it used to be, it may be time to get your eyes examined again because the prescription can change over time or you may have developed a new condition that may require treatment. You should call to schedule an appointment immediately if you have more serious symptoms including new floaters, flashes of light, or a dark curtain in your visual field.

Children younger than 9 years of age may develop a lazy eye (or amblyopia) if they have untreated refractive errors, including unequal or extreme nearsightedness. You should have your child examined by an eye doctor if he or she fails a vision screen at the pediatrician's office or at school.

Treatment • Most nearsightedness is treated with corrective lenses such as glasses or contact lenses. Some patients who are unable to tolerate or are unhappy with glasses or contact lenses may be eligible for refractive surgery such as LASIK (see chapter 4). You should talk with your eye doctor to find out more information.

Prognosis: Will I See Better? • The majority of people with myopia have excellent vision with appropriate treatment. Children with refractive amblyopia tend to have more successful outcomes if treated earlier.

Additional Resource

https://eyewiki.aao.org/Myopia

Farsightedness

BRAIN STAGG, MD AND PRATAP CHALLA, MD

What Is It? • Farsightedness, or hyperopia, is a condition in which distant objects are usually seen clearly but objects up close are blurred. Just as a camera uses lenses to properly focus light on film, the human eye uses the cornea and the lens to focus images on the retina. In farsightedness, the image that falls on the retina is blurred because the light entering the eye is focused behind the retina instead of directly on it. Farsightedness is caused by a cornea that is flatter than normal, a lens in the eye that is not strong enough, or an eyeball that is shorter than average. Approximately 25% of the general population is farsighted.

Many infants are born farsighted but lose their farsightedness by their teenage years. Children and young adults with mild or moderate hyperopia are often able to see clearly because their natural lens can change its shape, or accommodate, to focus on near objects. As farsighted people get older, however, their ability to accommodate declines as the lens becomes less flexible. Eventually, glasses or contact lenses may be required to correct their farsightedness.

Symptoms: What You May Experience • In adults, the vision is blurred at near but may be clearer at distance. You may notice eye strain or fatigue, especially when reading. A farsighted child who is not wearing glasses or contact lenses may not notice any difficulty seeing up close because of accommodation, but in some farsighted children, eye crossing (strabismus) may occur.

Examination Findings: What the Doctor Looks For • The eye doctor will test your vision and your need for glasses (refraction). In children, the pupils may also be dilated with eyedrops so that when refraction is performed, the eyes will not automatically adjust their focus. Note that farsightedness is rarely diagnosed in school vision screenings, which typically only test the ability to see distant objects.

What You Can Do • There is no proven way to prevent farsightedness from developing.

When to Call the Doctor • If you notice blurry vision at near but not at a distance, eye strain, or eye fatigue, you should call your eye doctor. Children with eye crossing or difficulty tracking objects up close should also promptly see an eye doctor and should have a dilated eye examination to rule out other eye problems. Even without vision complaints, children should have an eye exam at least once by the age of six to diagnose farsightedness or other eye conditions.

Treatment • Treating farsightedness depends on several factors, including your age and daily activities. Younger patients may or may not require glasses or contact lenses, depending on their ability to compensate for their farsightedness with accommodation. Older patients often benefit from glasses or contact lenses, which may only be necessary for reading if their farsightedness is mild. Some farsighted adults may benefit from refractive surgery, such as LASIK (see chapter 4), as another treatment option.

Prognosis: Will I See Better? • Most farsightedness can be fully corrected with glasses or contact lenses.

Additional Resource

https://eyewiki.aao.org/Hyperopia

Astigmatism

ONYEMAECHI NWANAJI-ENWEREM, MS AND PRIYATHAM S. METTU, MD

What Is It? • Astigmatism is an irregular curvature of the corneal surface of the eye. Instead of being spherical, like a basketball, the corneal surface is longer in certain axes, like a football. In eyes with astigmatism, light rays that enter the eye are focused unevenly, resulting in blurred vision at all distances. Most people have some degree of astigmatism, but severe cases can be associated with corneal diseases such as keratoconus or corneal scarring.

Symptoms: What You May Experience • You might notice that your vision is blurred or distorted when looking at objects either near or far without glasses or contact lenses. In some cases, astigmatism can contribute to headaches or eyestrain.

Examination Findings: What the Doctor Looks For • Your eye doctor will check your vision by having you look through various lenses with different powers to determine your glasses prescription and whether your glasses prescription includes any astigmatism. This is part of the standard comprehensive eye exam.

What You Can Do • There is generally no way to prevent astigmatism. However, if you have a corneal disease, such as keratoconus, then treating the underlying condition can prevent your astigmatism from getting worse.

When to Call the Doctor • People with blurry or distorted vision should be seen by an eye doctor to identify the condition and exclude nearsightedness or farsightedness, which can occur in combination with astigmatism.

Treatment • Astigmatism can usually be corrected with eyeglasses or contact lenses, including soft toric, gas-permeable, or hard contact lenses. In some cases, astigmatism can also be corrected by refractive surgery, such

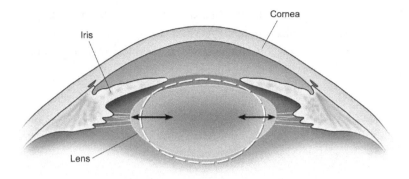
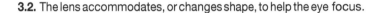

3.2. The lens accommodates, or changes shape, to help the eye focus.

as LASIK (see chapter 4), which aims to reshape the curve of the cornea. Irregular astigmatism caused by advanced keratoconus or corneal scarring may require more involved surgery such as a corneal transplant.

Prognosis: Will I See Better? • Most astigmatism can be fully corrected with eyeglasses or contact lenses, resulting in clearer vision.

Additional Resource

https://eyewiki.aao.org/Physiology_of_Astigmatism

Presbyopia

ONYEMAECHI NWANAJI-ENWEREM, MS AND PRIYATHAM S. METTU, MD

What Is It? • Presbyopia is a decrease in the ability to focus on near objects (arm's length or closer). It is a natural and expected part of the aging process. Normally, muscle fibers attached to the lens contract to alter the shape of the lens, allowing near objects to come into focus. This is called accommodation. As you age, the lens thickens and becomes stiff, decreasing its ability to change shape and leaving near vision out of focus. As a result, you may need reading glasses.

Symptoms: What You May Experience • As you reach middle age (around age 40–48), you will likely start to experience blurry vision when attempting to read fine print, and you may find that you have to hold reading materials farther away to see them clearly. Additional symptoms may include eyestrain or headache.

Examination Findings: What the Doctor Looks For • Presbyopia is readily detected as part of a standard eye exam. Your eye doctor may test the ability of each eye to accommodate for near vision by bringing an object closer and closer to the eye until the vision blurs.

What You Can Do • As it is a normal part of aging, all adults can expect to develop presbyopia. It is not preventable; however, certain systemic conditions and medications can increase the risk of developing presbyopia prematurely.

When to Call the Doctor • Presbyopia typically becomes most apparent during the mid-40s. It may occur at a slightly younger age for farsighted people or at an older age for those that are nearsighted. You should see an eye doctor when you notice that you are having trouble reading or performing near tasks comfortably.

Treatment • Presbyopia can typically be corrected with eyeglasses, which include reading glasses, bifocals, and progressive addition lenses, or with multifocal contact lenses. Over-the-counter reading glasses are an option for those who do not usually wear glasses to see far away or for those who wear distance contact lenses. Nearsighted individuals may find that they can take off their glasses to read and see up close, while still requiring glasses for distance vision.

Prognosis: Will I See Better? • Eyeglasses and contact lenses can usually fully correct presbyopia. However, you may need a more powerful reading prescription as you grow older.

Additional Resource
https://eyewiki.aao.org/Presbyopia

4 · Options for Correcting Vision

Eyeglasses

MICHELLE SY GO, MS, MD

Eyeglasses are the most common treatment for refractive error. Glasses work by changing the way light bends within the eye. In nearsightedness, the image is focused too far in front of the retina. A concave (inward curving) lens in the glasses is used to decrease the bend of light as it enters the eye. The resulting image is focused a little farther away and closer to the retina. In farsightedness and presbyopia, a convex (outward curving) lens is used to increase the amount that the entering light rays are bent. This brings the image more forward and closer to the retina. An eye with astigmatism and the lenses that correct it can be thought of as cylinders. A cylinder has one direction (or axis) that is very steep and another direction that is flat. An astigmatic lens can be positioned so that its steep axis corresponds with the flat axis of the eye. This causes all the directions of light from an image to be focused on the retina.

There can be 1 to 4 numbers in a prescription; you may only have one number if you do not have astigmatism or presbyopia. Take the example "−2.00 +1.00x90, add +2.50." The first number represents the sphere of the lens (−2.00 diopters); the second is astigmatism (+1.00 diopter); the third is the axis of astigmatism (90 degrees). A diopter is a unit of refractive power. For those with presbyopia, there is a fourth number (+2.50 diopters in the example above), which is called the "add" power, and is the additional power of lens needed at the bottom of the glasses for reading and seeing up close. It is important that the plus and minus signs in your glasses prescription are clearly written. Changing a plus to a minus sign can make a big difference, and vice versa. Additionally, the two eyes may have a different prescription.

If a prescription has add power, you can decide if you want to single vision glasses, bifocals, trifocals, or progressive lenses. Single vision means that you have one pair of eyeglasses for distance and a separate pair of glasses for near vision. Glasses other than single vision have more than

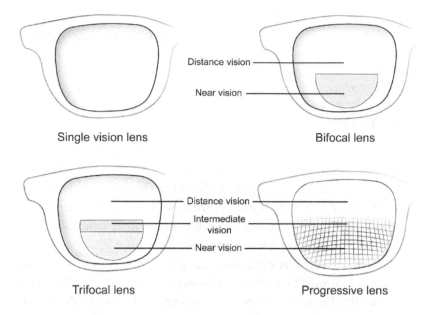

Single vision lens

Distance vision

Near vision

Bifocal lens

Distance vision

Intermediate vision

Near vision

Trifocal lens

Progressive lens

4.1. Top left: single-vision glasses lens. Top right: bifocal glasses lens. Bottom left: trifocal glasses lens. Bottom right: progressive glasses lens.

one prescription ground into the lens. A bifocal lens is made so that the top part of the lens has the distance prescription and the bottom part has the near correction. A trifocal lens has an additional middle lens for intermediate distance. A progressive lens is made so that there is a gradual progression of the power as you go down the lens, with distance at the top and reading at the bottom, and no visible line in the lens separating each prescription change.

There are many options regarding lens material, shape, and treatments. Glass lenses, which are heavier and more fragile than plastic lenses, are no longer commonly used. Most eyeglasses nowadays are made of plastic. High-index plastic lenses have the added benefit of being thinner and more lightweight, and offer 100% ultraviolet (uv) protection compared to traditional plastic lenses. Polycarbonate and trivex lenses are the recommended lenses for protective eyewear as these materials are shatter resistant. They also naturally block uv light and are even more lightweight than high-index lenses. An option for lens shape is the aspheric lens, which is thinner and flatter than the typical lens. Since a high-powered lens tends to make your eyes appear bigger (high plus) or smaller (high minus) to others looking at you, an aspheric lens can minimize this undesired effect and also improve optical quality. There are even more options when it comes to lens enhancements such as antireflective, antiscratch, and uv-blocking coatings. Photochromic treatment, commonly referred to as transition lenses, is a popular lens upgrade where the lens becomes tinted in sunlight. Choosing the right frame is also important as it can affect your appearance, comfort, and vision. Talk to your optician to determine which of these many options are best for your needs.

Additional Resource

https://www.aao.org/eye-health/glasses-contacts/glasses

Contact Lenses

MICHELLE SY GO, MS, MD

Contact lenses are a popular alternative to eyeglasses and refractive surgery for the correction of nearsightedness, farsightedness, astigmatism, and even presbyopia. People who play sports, have high refractive error or irregular astigmatism, or who want to be spectacle independent can potentially benefit from contact lenses. There are also special types of contact lenses for treating medical conditions. These include scleral contact lenses for keratoconus and other corneal diseases, prosthetic lenses for improving the appearance of injured or abnormally shaped eyes, and bandage contact lenses for managing corneal defects or leaks after surgery. This chapter will focus on contact lenses, which correct refractive error.

The two main types of contact lenses are soft and hard. Hard contacts are also known as rigid gas permeable contacts. As the name suggests, soft lenses are made of pliable plastic material that conforms to the front surface of the eye. Nowadays, they are most commonly made of silicone hydrogel, which allows more oxygen to reach the cornea. Rigid gas permeable lenses are made out of stiffer, durable plastic; it may take longer to get used to how they feel compared to soft lenses. In exchange, hard lenses address a wider range of refractive errors and can offer better quality vision.

Another way to categorize contact lenses is by wearing time and replacement frequency. Daily contact lenses must be removed every night.

Extended-wear and continuous-wear contact lenses are approved by the Food and Drug Administration (FDA) to be worn overnight and up to a few days to a month depending on the brand. You should always follow the appropriate replacement schedule for your contact lenses. Daily disposable lenses need to be replaced every day, while other types of soft lenses should be discarded every 2 weeks, monthly, or longer according to the instructions. Rigid gas permeable lenses have the greatest longevity and may not need to be replaced for a year or longer.

Contact lens design varies based on the refractive error that is being corrected. A spherical soft contact lens has the same power over the entire lens and can correct nearsightedness or farsightedness. Options for astigmatic correction include toric soft contacts, hard contacts, or hybrid contacts. Lenses made with add power to correct presbyopia are known as multifocal contact lenses. Cosmetic, or decorative, contact lenses are used for their appearance rather than their visual correction. Buying these lenses without a prescription from a beauty supply store or other novelty store can put you at risk of serious complications such as eye infection, loss of vision, and even loss of the eye. You should only purchase FDA-approved contact lenses from a reputable source with a proper contact lens prescription.

After you get your contact lenses, you must care for them appropriately. Daily disposable contact lenses do not require cleaning because they are discarded after each use. Other types of lenses can be cleaned and disinfected with multipurpose or preservative-free solutions such as those that contain some hydrogen peroxide. You should never wash your contact lenses with homemade saline, tap water, or saliva. If you develop eye discomfort, redness, decreased vision, or eye pain with contact lens use, you should discontinue contact lens use and call your eye doctor immediately.

Additional Resources

https://www.aao.org/eye-health/glasses-contacts/contact-lens-types
https://www.allaboutvision.com/contacts/contact_lenses.htm

Refractive Surgery

CASSANDRA C. BROOKS, MD AND PREEYA GUPTA, MD

What Is Refractive Surgery? • Refractive surgery, or vision correction surgery, is a group of procedures aimed at reducing or potentially eliminating reliance on glasses or contact lenses. There are a variety of techniques, the most common of which is laser, to achieve this goal. LASIK (laser-assisted in situ keratomileusis) and PRK (photorefractive keratectomy) are the most commonly performed laser refractive procedures. Radial keratotomy (RK), a procedure where small cuts are made in the cornea, is no longer commonly performed. LASIK surgery can be used to treat nearsightedness, farsightedness, and astigmatism. A flap is created in the cornea using one type of laser and then a second laser is used to reshape the cornea to correct for the refractive error (glasses prescription). Similar to LASIK, PRK is used to treat nearsightedness, farsightedness, and astigmatism. Unlike LASIK, there is no corneal flap used in PRK. The surface cells of the cornea are removed and then a laser treatment reshapes the cornea to correct the refractive error. A contact lens is placed for 5–7 days while the surface epithelial cells heal. Recovery from PRK is typically longer than with LASIK, but final visual potential is the same.

Who Might Consider Refractive Surgery? • Individuals interested in reducing or eliminating their dependence on glasses or contact lenses are potential candidates for refractive surgery. Some may be looking to improve their visual quality of life, while others may find glasses or contact lenses a potential hazard given their environment (e.g., toxic chemicals, dirty, or dusty worksites) or profession (e.g., law enforcement, firefighter, athlete). If you are considering refractive surgery, make an appointment with an ophthalmologist to determine if you are a good candidate. An ophthalmologist will take into account your age, glasses prescription, other eye and systemic diseases, corneal imaging, and goals of surgery to determine if refractive surgery is the right choice for you.

In general, good candidates must have a stable glasses prescription for at least 1 year and, for consideration of LASIK, must be over the age of 21 (per the Food and Drug Administration unless special circumstances exist). There is no upper age limit, although as you approach your mid-50s, you naturally start the development of cataracts, which would not be treated appropriately with laser vision correction. If you have a history of ocular herpes infections, rheumatoid arthritis, systemic lupus erythematous or other diseases that may impede corneal healing, then you may not be a good candidate for refractive surgery. An ophthalmologist will also examine and measure your cornea to determine if the corneal thickness is sufficient to safely remove the amount of tissue needed to treat the refractive error. Before your appointment and prior to obtaining corneal measurements, you must not wear soft contact lenses for at least 2 weeks in order to achieve the most accurate eye measurements. If you wear toric or rigid gas permeable contact lenses, they need to be out of your eyes for an even longer period in order to obtain accurate corneal measurements.

Although there are many refractive surgeries available, every procedure is not ideal for everyone. Patients who are good candidates still need to take into consideration the postoperative limitations and potential risks involved with surgery as well as maintain reasonable expectations regarding results.

How Does Refractive Surgery Work? • LASIK, the most common type of refractive surgery, works by reshaping the cornea (the clear front surface of the eye) in order to change the focusing power of the eye. Refractive surgery begins with multiple precise measurements of the eye to develop a surgical plan tailored to your anatomy and refractive error. During surgery, two separate lasers are used, one to create the flap on the corneal surface and one to reshape the underlying corneal tissue. The laser reshapes the cornea by removing very thin layers (microns) of tissue in a precise fashion. PRK is similar; however rather than creating a corneal flap, the surface corneal cells are simply removed and allowed to heal after the procedure.

A modern advancement in laser vision correction is wavefront technology. This technology can be thought of as taking a fingerprint-like map of the cornea to allow the surgeon to tailor the laser treatment to your eye and treat higher-order visual aberrations. Higher-order aberrations are tiny optical imperfections that distort image quality and are not correctable with glasses or contact lenses. During surgery, wavefront technology can be used to smooth out these imperfections, leaving you with the best possible vision.

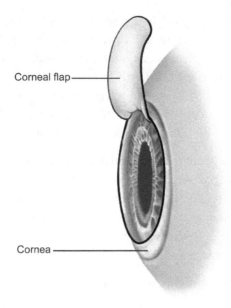

Corneal flap ⎯⎯⎯⎯

Cornea ⎯⎯⎯⎯⎯⎯⎯

4.2. A flap is made in the cornea during LASIK surgery.

If your cornea is too thin or the corneal map is too irregular, a phakic intraocular lens implant is an option. In this procedure, a corrective lens is placed into the eye behind the iris but in front of the natural lens. It can be thought of as an implantable contact lens which provides vision correction. This procedure is more invasive than laser surgery, however it is reversible. Currently in the United States, implantable contact lenses are only indicated to treat nearsightedness and astigmatism.

What Are the Risks of Refractive Surgery? • For the appropriate candidate, laser vision corrective surgery is a safe and effective procedure. However, it is important to recognize that not everyone is a good surgical candidate and no surgery is completely risk free. During your consultation with an ophthalmologist, the risks involved in surgery should be reviewed. Since laser procedures can cause or worsen dry eye symptoms, those who already have dry eyes may not be a good surgical candidate. Overall, there is a 1–2% chance of a "minor" complication, which may slow your recovery, result in a small visual disturbance, or require additional procedures to address. There is an up-to 0.4% chance of a "major" complication, which may permanently reduce your vision. Follow-up after surgery is very important to monitor for any complications so that any potential issues can be addressed early.

It is important to recognize that refractive surgery does not correct cataracts, glaucoma, or age-related macular degeneration, therefore continued follow-up for these conditions is recommended.

How Long Do the Results of Refractive Surgery Last? • For the vast majority, the results of refractive surgery are long lasting. Laser correction of nearsightedness tends to last longer than correction of farsightedness. Overall, about 6–8% will require additional correction in the future, known as "enhancement," to maintain excellent vision. If you experience changes in vision, you should seek care from an ophthalmologist.

What Other Factors Are Important When Considering Refractive Surgery? • It is important to do your research and find a qualified, experienced ophthalmologist and facility when considering refractive surgery. If you are contemplating eye surgery, then undergoing surgery at a facility with high-quality staff, technology, and service will provide the best long-term results.

Additional Resources

https://www.aao.org/eye-health/treatments/what-is-refractive-surgery
https://eyewiki.aao.org/LASIK_for_Myopia_and_Astigmatism%3A_Safety
    _and_Efficacy
https://eyewiki.aao.org/Photorefractive_Keratectomy

Protective Eyewear

MICHELLE SY GO, MS, MD

Eye injuries are alarmingly common at home and in the workplace. It is estimated that more than 2,000 people experience an eye injury at work every day and that proper eye protection could have prevented or lessened the severity of the injury in about 90% of cases. The type of protective eyewear should be appropriate for the task at hand. In general, you should wear glasses with side shields for activities that involve dust and flying particles. Use goggles when working with chemicals or if there is risk of splash injury (there should also be eyewash stations at your workplace if you commonly work with hazardous chemicals). Welding and laser devices emit radiation and require special safety glasses for welding and for each type of laser. Regular safety glasses do not provide adequate protection from welding or laser injuries.

The lenses in the protective eyewear can be classified as basic or high impact according to American National Standards Institute (ANSI). Basic impact means there are no cracks or breaks when a 1-inch steel ball is dropped from a height of 50 inches onto the lens. High impact means that the lens and frame remain intact when a ¼-inch steel ball is shot toward the lens at 150 feet per second. If you see a "+" mark on the glasses, it means they have passed the high impact test. Shaded glasses may display a number representing optical density (related to how much light is transmitted through the lens), ranging from 1.5 to 14 with higher numbers indicating a darker lens. Most lenses are made of polycarbonate, which is lighter and more impact-resistant than glass.

Frames also undergo a similar assessment to differentiate basic impact from high impact frames as well as to indicate durability testing. ANSI-compliant frames are marked with "Z87" for basic impact and "Z87+" for high impact. Safety glasses can also be made with basic or high impact prescription lenses and the corresponding frames will be marked with "Z87–2." If you are unsure which safety glasses to purchase, choose high impact resistant lenses and frames for the most protection.

Safety glasses are also important for sports. High impact safety glasses with a wrap-around frame are recommended for activities such as hunting, shooting, and fishing. You may consider an antireflective coating or polarized tint to reduce glare. If you play paintball or handball, you should always wear a helmet or a head shield whenever you are in the play area. Call your eye doctor or go to the nearest emergency department immediately if you have had an eye injury.

Additional Resources

https://www.preventblindness.org/eye-safety-work
https://www.aao.org/eye-health/tips-prevention/injuries-protective-eyewear

Blepharitis

CHARLENE L. JAMES, OD

What Is It? • Blepharitis is inflammation of the eyelid margin, where the eyelashes start, and is a common cause of ocular discomfort and irritation. It usually affects both eyes and may be characterized as "anterior blepharitis" or "posterior blepharitis," although they are often present simultaneously. In anterior blepharitis, hard scales and crusting form at the base of the eyelashes as a reaction to certain bacteria that live there. Long-standing cases may result in eyelash loss, eyelashes that turn in, or scarring at the base of the eyelashes. Posterior blepharitis affects the oil glands, called meibomian glands, located at the base of the eyelashes. Normally, the meibomian glands produce a clear, thin fluid which coats the front surface of the eye and helps keep the eye lubricated. However, when these glands become inflamed, the oily secretions become thickened and eventually stop flowing completely.

Symptoms: What You May Experience • The symptoms of anterior and posterior blepharitis are similar in that both conditions cause irritation, burning, and light sensitivity. Redness and crusting at the base of the eyelashes is also common. Symptoms are usually worse in the morning, although you may notice an increase in symptoms during the day.

Examination Findings: What the Doctor Looks For • If you have this condition, your eye doctor will be able to identify hard scales and crusting mainly located around the base of the eyelashes. Your eye doctor can also identify abnormal meibomian gland secretions at the base of the eyelashes, which will appear as oil plugs blocking the pores of the glands. The cornea and conjunctiva will be examined for signs of irritation or dry eye.

What You Can Do • Apply warm compresses for several minutes to your eyelids twice per day to soften the crusting at the base of the eyelashes. Cleanse your lids to mechanically remove crusting twice per day with a 50:50 solution of baby shampoo and water on a washcloth or cotton ball. Commercially produced soap pads for lid scrubs are available over the counter. Preservative-free artificial tear drops, which are also available over the counter, can be used for symptoms of burning, irritation, and redness. Once the condition has improved, lid hygiene can be performed less frequently. However, the condition will eventually return if lid cleansing is stopped completely.

When to Call the Doctor • You should consult with your eye doctor if you have been doing warm compresses and lid cleansing for several weeks at home and are not improving. Your condition may require additional prescription medications, which only an eye doctor may provide.

Treatment • In cases where warm compresses and lid cleansing fail to control symptoms, treatment with antibiotics may be necessary. Oral antibiotics, typically azithromycin or doxycycline, may be used for several weeks to treat more severe cases of blepharitis. Erythromycin ointment may be used in children. Preservative-free artificial tears may also be helpful in soothing an irritated eye.

Prognosis: Will I See Better? • With proper treatment and maintenance, the prognosis for this condition is very good. Once a lid hygiene regimen is established, regular maintenance as a part of a daily routine can keep this condition controlled. Lid hygiene is important as it not only improves irritation, but also prevents blepharitis from causing other problems such as dry eye, styes, and discomfort with contact lens wear. It is important to remember, however, that having this condition will require a long-term lid hygiene regimen to keep symptoms at bay.

Additional Resources
https://www.aao.org/eye-health/diseases/blepharitis-treatment
https://eyewiki.aao.org/Blepharitis

Ocular Rosacea

CHARLENE L. JAMES, OD

What Is It? • Rosacea is an inflammatory condition of the skin that affects the face, chest, and eyes. The exact cause of rosacea is unknown, but it may be associated with heredity and environmental factors such as excessive sun exposure. Rosacea usually affects people between the ages of 30 and 50, and women are more prone to the disease than men.

When rosacea affects the eyes, it is called "ocular rosacea." Ocular rosacea causes inflammation of the oil glands in the eyelids and can lead to blepharitis, styes, and ocular surface irritation. Surface irritation of the eye can lead to other inflammatory conditions such as conjunctivitis, corneal ulcers, episcleritis, and uveitis. Surface irritation of the eye can also cause new abnormal blood vessels to grow into the normally clear cornea, resulting in scarring and even decreased vision.

Symptoms: What You May Experience • You may experience eye irritation, burning, redness, and excessive tearing if affected by ocular rosacea. You may also feel like there is sand or grit in your eye, have blurred vision, or develop more frequent styes. The skin on your face may appear flushed, especially when drinking alcohol or hot beverages. In the long-term, rosacea may cause thickened skin and enlargement of the nose.

Examination Findings: What the Doctor Looks For • Signs of ocular rosacea include flushed complexion, abnormal blood vessels on the eyelids, and adult acne. Signs of blepharitis on your eyelids is common with ocular rosacea, along with chronic irritation or inflammation of the front surface of the eye. Your eye doctor will be able to identify these signs of inflammation during the examination.

What You Can Do • There is no proven way to prevent the occurrence or development of rosacea. A lid-hygiene regimen including warm compresses to the closed eyelids, eyelid cleansing with a 50:50 mixture of baby shampoo and water twice daily, and the use of preservative-free artificial tears as needed will help alleviate symptoms of ocular rosacea.

When to Call the Doctor • If your eye irritation is not improved with a regular lid-hygiene regimen and artificial tears, you should contact your eye doctor. You should also contact your eye doctor with any signs of abnormal facial flushing or adult acne. Decreased vision or eye discharge could be signs of a severe eye problem and you should see your eye doctor right away.

Treatment • In addition to artificial tears and lid hygiene, ocular rosacea is usually treated with low-dose oral antibiotics, such as doxycycline, over several weeks or months. These low-dose antibiotics are used not only for their antibacterial properties, but also to reduce inflammation of the oil glands. Ask your doctor about the risks of taking oral antibiotics for a long period of time. If irritation and surface inflammation is severe, topical steroid eye drops may be prescribed as well.

Prognosis: Will I See Better? • Rosacea is a chronic condition that requires ongoing treatment. Treatments aim to control inflammation of the skin and oil glands, leading to improvement in symptoms. A daily maintenance regimen of warm compresses, artificial tears, and oral antibiotics or other eye drops (if prescribed) will help keep symptoms at bay and your eyes feeling comfortable.

Additional Resource
https://eyewiki.aao.org/Ocular_Rosacea

Stye and Chalazion

KIRIN KHAN, MD

What Is It? • A stye, also known as a hordeolum, is a type of eyelid infection that occurs when one of the oil (meibomian) glands of the eyelid becomes blocked. Bacteria within the blocked gland cause an infection resulting in a swollen, red bump on the eyelid. Styes can occur on either the upper or lower eyelid and on either the outside or inside of the eyelid. Internal styes tend to be more painful.

Chalazia are caused by complete blockage of one of the glands of the eyelid. In contrast to styes, chalazia are not an infection, but rather an inflammatory reaction. The eyelid nodule in this condition is less red and painful. A chalazion can follow a stye when the bacteria in the blocked gland are cleared by the body but the gland continues to be clogged. Chalazia tend to persist longer than styes. Individuals with an ocular condition known as blepharitis are at higher risk for developing both styes and chalazia.

Symptoms: What You May Experience • A stye will be a red, swollen, and painful bump on either the inside or outside of the eyelid. The infection develops over a period of days and is similar in appearance to a pimple. Occasionally, the infection can extend past the singular eyelid nodule to cause redness, pain, and swelling in the entire eyelid, cheek, or other areas of the face (called cellulitis). Additional symptoms include tearing of the affected eye, a gritty sensation in the eye, sensitivity to light, and general eyelid tenderness.

A chalazion will present as a firm, painless nodule on the eyelid. Chalazia develop over a longer period and last longer than styes. Additionally, when compared to styes, chalazia tend to be less red and swollen. Rarely, a large chalazion can press on the surface of the eyeball resulting in distortion of the eye's shape, known as astigmatism, which causes blurry vision.

Examination Findings: What the Doctor Looks For • Both styes and chalazia can be diagnosed on a clinical exam conducted by an eye doctor. The eye doctor will examine the eyelids for any bumps or nodules, paying special attention to redness, swelling, and tenderness. To facilitate the diagnosis of an internal eyelid bump, the physician may have to flip the eyelids to see the underside of the eyelid. There are no special tests required in the diagnosis of either of these two conditions.

What You Can Do • Prevention of styes and chalazia begins with good eyelid hygiene. In general, you should only touch the eyes with clean, washed hands. Safe eye makeup routines, including not using makeup beyond its expiration date and not sharing eye makeup with others, can also help reduce the incidence of these conditions. Similarly, contact lenses should be handled in a hygienic way. Individuals with blepharitis or those prone to styes and chalazia should clean the lash line with diluted baby shampoo or cleansing pads nightly.

Warm compresses can be used to treat styes or chalazia at home. This involves wetting a clean cloth with warm water and holding the cloth with gentle pressure against the affected eyelid. When the cloth cools, wet it again with warm water. Repeat this process for 10–15 minutes four times a day. Pushing, squeezing, or popping an eyelid bump is not recommended and can worsen the condition. Individuals with a stye or chalazion should discontinue use of eye makeup and contact lenses until the condition resolves.

When to Call the Doctor • A stye should resolve within 1–2 weeks of onset. Chalazia persist longer but should resolve within a month of onset. Contact your eye doctor if these conditions persist longer than expected or worsen despite treatment. Additionally, consult an eye doctor if an eyelid bump causes severe vision changes or if the redness and swelling extends past a singular bump to include larger areas, such as the eye, entire eyelid, cheek, or other portions of the face. Seek attention if an eyelid bump begins to bleed or if it is accompanied by fever. Recurring eyelid nodules warrant attention by an ophthalmologist as they can be a sign of a serious but rare type of skin cancer that arises from the sebaceous glands.

Treatment • First-line treatment for styes and chalazia include warm compresses as described above. Persistent styes can be treated in the office by an ophthalmologist by incision and drainage of the bump, which involves opening the stye and allowing the blocked contents to be released. Styes with redness and swelling that extend to include larger portions of the face will require oral antibiotics. The doctor may prescribe topical antibiotics or ointment to apply to the eyelid after treating the stye. Persistent chalazia may be treated with an injection of steroid into the nodule or surgical removal of the nodule.

Prognosis: Will I See Better? • Styes and chalazia have an excellent prognosis. Most styes will resolve within days to weeks with use of warm compresses as described above. Chalazia tend to persist longer but also have a high likelihood of clearing without intervention by a physician. Styes or chalazia that require medical intervention also tend to heal quite well without causing any lasting vision changes.

Additional Resources

https://eyewiki.aao.org/Stye

https://eyewiki.org/Chalazion

https://www.aao.org/eye-health/diseases/what-are-chalazia-styes

Dacryocystitis: Infection of the Tear Drainage Pathway

LEON RAFAILOV, MD

What Is It? • Dacryocystitis is an infection of the tear drainage system, which is located on the upper part of the nose and inner part of the eye. Tears are normally made by the lacrimal gland located under the lateral side of the upper eyelid. Tears then drain out through a system of ducts in the eyelid to the lacrimal sac and out into the nose (this is why you have a runny nose when you cry). If there is a blockage in this drainage system, tears cannot drain and bacteria can grow within the duct or lacrimal sac causing dacryocystitis. Dacryocystitis can be acute with rapid swelling and pain over a few days, or chronic, lasting weeks to months. Blockage of the tear drainage system may be due to aging, injury, sinus disease, inflammatory disease, a mass in the lacrimal system or nose, or scarring from previous episodes of dacryocystitis. In severe cases, the infection can spread to the surrounding skin and other areas of the face or eye socket (called cellulitis), which requires immediate medical attention.

Symptoms: What You May Experience • Tears constantly flow from the lacrimal gland, lubricate the surface of the eyeball, and drain out through the tear ducts and lacrimal sac into the nose. If you have a blockage in your tear drainage system, you may notice excessive tearing of your eyes. If an infection develops, you may notice redness, pain, warmth, and swelling of the skin below the inner corner of the eye and upper part of the nose. The eye itself may also feel irritated.

Examination Findings: What the Doctor Looks For • Your eye doctor will examine the area where the tear drainage system is located, just below the inner corner of the eye. The doctor may press on the area to see if purulent material can be expressed as well as try to irrigate the tear drainage system with a small cannula to check for a blockage.

What You Can Do • If you notice pain, redness, and/or swelling of the area of skin just below the inner corner of the eye, apply warm compresses frequently and call your eye doctor promptly.

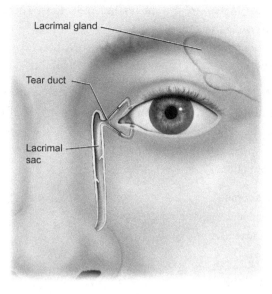

Lacrimal gland

Tear duct

Lacrimal sac

5.1. Tears flow from the lacrimal gland, lubricate the surface of the eyeball, and drain through the tear ducts and lacrimal sac into the nose.

When to Call the Doctor • If you develop constant, excessive tearing, see your ophthalmologist, because a blockage of the tear duct system can be treated before an infection develops. Once you notice pain, redness, warmth, and/or swelling of the skin below the inner corner of the eye, see your eye doctor promptly so treatment can be started before the infection spreads.

Treatment • Active dacryocystitis is treated with oral antibiotics and antibiotic eye drops. Warm compresses can help the infection resolve faster. If the infection has already spread to the surrounding areas of the face, then intravenous antibiotics and hospitalization may be needed. If an abscess develops, the doctor may need to create a small skin incision to allow the pus to drain out. Once the active infection is controlled and inflammation is reduced, you may be a candidate for surgery to open the tear drainage system to prevent further infections. This operation is called dacryocystorhinostomy (DCR) and is performed in the operating room, often under general anesthesia. In a DCR, a direct passage for tears is created between the lacrimal sac and the inside of the nose.

Prognosis: Will I See Better? • Most cases of dacryocystitis resolve with antibiotic treatment. Because the infection is caused by a blocked tear duct in most cases, dacryocystitis often recurs if the blockage is not treated. Surgery to open up the tear drainage system will fix the blockage in over 90% of patients.

Additional Resources

https://www.healthline.com/health/dacryocystitis
https://eyewiki.aao.org/Dacryocystitis

Drooping Eyelids

LEON RAFAILOV, MD

What Is It? • Drooping upper eyelids, known as ptosis (pronounced toe-sis), can occur at birth, or more commonly in adulthood. Newborns with ptosis (congenital ptosis) usually have an underdeveloped muscle that lifts the upper eyelid, while adult ptosis can have a variety of causes. The most common cause for adult ptosis is age-related loosening of the muscle that lifts the upper eyelid. Injury, muscle diseases, or nerve diseases are also potential causes of ptosis. Many often develop ptosis after eye surgery, yet this does not necessarily indicate that something went wrong during the surgery, but rather may be a consequence of necessary manipulation of the eyelid at the time of surgery.

Besides being a cosmetic problem, drooping upper eyelids can block upward vision and even central vision in severe cases. If the ptosis is the result of a nerve problem, this can indicate a more serious neurologic disease that needs to be evaluated as it can impact your general health. In infants, drooping upper eyelids can cause amblyopia (poor visual development) by blocking vision or causing astigmatism, which distorts the vision. Infants will often need to be checked by an eye doctor to see if the child is at risk for amblyopia.

Symptoms: What You May Experience • If your upper eyelids droop, you may notice that your eyelids block your vision when you look upward or even straight ahead. You may have trouble reading, because your eyelids may droop even more when you are looking down. Some people may develop tension headaches from raising their eyebrows all day to compensate for droopy eyelids. Let your doctor know if the degree of ptosis fluctuates throughout the day (often becoming much worse later in the day). Also, let your doctor know if you have double vision, difficulty swallowing or breathing, or changes to the size of your pupil as this may reflect a more serious neurological cause of your ptosis.

Examination Findings: What the Doctor Looks For • Your eye doctor will ask questions about how long your upper eyelids have drooped and if the droopiness fluctuates, as well as if you have any muscle or nerve diseases. He or she will measure your eyelid position and test how far you can raise your upper eyelids and if you can close your eyelids completely. Your pupils and eye movements will be examined, since nerve damage that causes drooping eyelids can also affect these functions. Your peripheral vision may be checked with a machine to determine if your ptosis is blocking your upward field of view, and photographs showing your eyelid position may be taken. The doctor may put dilating drops in your eye to test if one of the muscles on the inside of the eyelid is still active as this may help them choose the best type of surgery to treat your condition.

What You Can Do • Besides avoiding injury to the upper eyelid and its muscle, there is no way to prevent ptosis from developing. If ptosis is present in your child, bring them to a pediatric eye doctor to make sure it is not impacting their vision during their critical visual development stage, otherwise a lazy eye (amblyopia) may develop.

When to Call the Doctor • If your upper eyelids droop and block your vision, see your ophthalmologist to discuss treatment options. An ophthalmologist should be seen promptly if the ptosis is present in an infant or child, is new or fluctuates, or is accompanied by unequal pupils or double vision. If the ptosis occurs along with new weakness in other muscles, or difficulty breathing, swallowing, or speaking, go to your local emergency room immediately as this may represent a serious neurological condition.

Treatment • The treatment of ptosis usually involves surgery in the operating room or minor procedure room to raise the eyelids. Your ophthalmologist will choose the best surgical technique depending on the amount of ptosis and the function of the muscle that lifts the upper eyelid. Most ptosis repairs are performed with numbing injections and sedation for comfort, although in rare cases general anesthesia may be necessary. General anesthesia is almost always necessary in surgery on young children. After surgery, you may temporarily have some trouble closing the eyelid, so it is very important to frequently use lubricating and antibiotic eyedrops and ointment as directed by your surgeon.

Prognosis: Will I See Better? • Most ptosis surgeries are successful, although it is often hard to get the eyelids perfectly symmetrical. Rarely, patients require more than one surgery to fully correct ptosis.

Additional Resources

https://www.aao.org/eye-health/diseases/what-is-ptosis
https://www.asoprs.org/droopy-eyelids—ptosis-
https://eyewiki.aao.org/Blepharoptosis

Ectropion and Entropion: Everted and Inverted Eyelids

LEON RAFAILOV, MD

What Is It? • Ectropion means an outward turning of the edge of the eyelid away from the eyeball. In most cases, it is the lower eyelid that is affected by ectropion. Ectropion usually occurs because the lower eyelid tissues relax with gravity as a person ages. Other causes of ectropion include nerve problems, scarring from sun damage or previous eyelid injury, or abnormal growths that pull the eyelid out of position. Ectropion can lead to tearing problems, as the eyelid needs to be pressed up against the eyeball in order for tears to drain properly. Ectropion can also lead to dryness of the eye surface as it does not allow the eyelid to properly close and lubricate the eye during blinking.

Entropion, on the other hand, is an inward turning of the edge of the eyelid toward the eyeball. As with ectropion, the lower eyelid is most commonly affected. Causes of entropion include aging, eyelid muscle spasms, scarring, and birth defects (in newborns). Most of the problems caused by entropion come from the eyelashes rubbing against the surface of the eyeball as the eyelid turns inward.

Symptoms: What You May Experience • With ectropion, you may see that your lower eyelid sags instead of resting tightly against the eyeball. This can lead to tearing, dryness, irritation and redness of the eye. In entropion, your lower eyelid may curl inward, toward your eyeballs, rubbing the eye as you blink. This scratching of the eye may cause irritation, burning and in severe cases, injury to the cornea causing cloudiness, scarring, and possible infection.

Examination Findings: What the Doctor Looks For • Your eye doctor will examine the position of your eyelids and look for a cause of the ectropion or entropion. Your doctor will assess the position of the tear drainage system opening in the lower eyelid and check to see if eyelashes are rubbing against your eye. Your eye doctor will also examine the surface of your eye for tear problems or for corneal damage.

What You Can Do • There is no proven way to avoid developing ectropion or entropion. If you have entropion and are waiting for your appointment, it may help to tape the eyelid downward to the cheek to help keep your eyelashes from scratching your eye.

When to Call the Doctor • If you notice that your eyelid turns inward or outward, or if you experience excessive watering/tearing of the eye, redness, irritation, or burning, then you should see your eye doctor.

Treatment • Treatment of ectropion and entropion depends on the underlying cause. If age and gravity have caused the lower eyelid to sag outward or turn inward, surgery is often indicated to tighten and restore the eyelid to its natural position. This type of surgery is usually performed in the operating room or the procedure room in a clinic with sedation and local numbing injections. Temporary treatments include lubricating eye drops and ointment and taping of the lower eyelid into a more normal position. If the ectropion is due to scarring, the surgeon may use a skin graft below your eyelid to help prop up the eyelid against the eyeball.

For entropion, treatments are often similar to the eyelid-tightening surgery in ectropion. Other treatments can include plucking inverted eyelashes or permanently destroying the inverted eyelashes by freezing or heating the base of those hair follicles.

Prognosis: Will I See Better? • The final outcome depends on the specific cause and extent of eyelid turning. Ectropion and entropion caused by scarring are more difficult to treat. Most cases of ectropion and entropion can be improved with minor surgery.

Additional Resources

https://www.asoprs.org/ectropion
https://www.asoprs.org/entropion

Cancers and Benign Lesions of the Eyelids

LEON RAFAILOV, MD

What Is It? • Growths on the eyelids can be divided into those that are cancerous and those that are benign (noncancerous). Benign eyelid growths are much more common, making up about 85% of all eyelid growths. Most of these growths come from the skin of the eyelid itself. While cancerous eyelid growths are rarer, it is important to recognize them early and have them treated promptly.

There are several types of cancer that occur on the eyelids. The most common variety (comprising 90–95% of eyelid cancers) is basal cell carcinoma, which arises from eyelid skin. Basal cell carcinoma can be located on the skin anywhere in the body, but it is usually found in sun-exposed areas. Squamous cell carcinoma also grows from eyelid skin, while sebaceous cell carcinoma is a rare cancer of the eyelid oil glands (also called sebaceous glands). Melanoma is a cancer of the pigmented cells in the skin. In general, the risk that an eyelid lesion is cancerous increases with a history of heavy sun exposure, immunosuppression, previous skin cancers, previous radiation, smoking, or a fair skin complexion.

Benign eyelid lesions, of which there are many types, can be cosmetically unsightly or irritating but pose less risk to your health. Some of these are precancerous, meaning they may progress to cancer in the future and may require closer monitoring after they are treated.

Symptoms: What You May Experience • You may see a growth on your eyelid, though often patients do not notice these growths themselves. Symptoms suggesting that a growth is cancerous include rapid growth, poor healing, irregular borders, bleeding and crusting of the lesion, color changes, a pearly appearance, changes in the shape of the eyelid margin or edge, loss of eyelashes, and abnormal blood vessels on the lesion.

Examination Findings: What the Doctor Looks For • Your eye doctor will examine your eyelid lesion and decide if there is a risk that it is cancerous. Some of the most important questions the doctor may ask would be about the growth and age of the lesion. If you have photos showing what it looked like before, bring them to your appointment so your doctor can compare.

What You Can Do • Many eyelid growths are not preventable, but you can reduce your risk of developing skin cancer by using sunscreen, avoiding excessive sun exposure, and not smoking.

When to Call the Doctor • You should see your eye doctor for any eyelid lesion that is bothersome. It is especially important to be examined promptly if the lesion is growing, bleeding, crusting, distorting the eyelid, changing color, or causing loss or change in color of the eyelashes as these are signs a lesion may be cancerous.

Treatment • When your eye doctor examines your eyelid lesion, they will decide if cancer is suspected. If the lesion appears small and benign, it can usually be removed in the office using a local anesthetic injection to numb the area before removal. You may require stitches and antibiotic ointment while it heals. If your ophthalmologist suspects an eyelid cancer, they will take a sample of the lesion and send it to the pathology laboratory to determine whether cancer is present and, if so, what type of cancer and whether the edges of the sample are cancer free. The pathology results may take several weeks to return. If the lesion is large or if the edges of the sample still contain cancer, more of the lesion will have to be removed. Your ophthalmologist may send you to see a highly trained dermatologist called a Mohs surgeon. Mohs micrographic surgery is a specialized way to remove cancerous skin cells that allows you to keep as much healthy skin as possible. Depending on the location and size of the lesion that is removed, you may be sent back to an oculoplastic surgeon within 1–2 days after Mohs surgery for closure and reconstruction of your eyelid.

Prognosis: Will I See Better? • Many eyelid growths, both cancerous and benign, are easily treated by removing them surgically. Larger or deeper growths are more difficult to remove because they may extend into critical portions of the eyelid and even rarely onto the eyeball itself. Basal cell carcinoma, which is the most common eyelid cancer, rarely spreads to other areas of the body and rarely grows back after it is removed. Other types of eyelid cancer may behave more aggressively and require chemotherapy or radiation in addition to surgery. Your doctor will need to see you regularly after your surgery to monitor for recurrence of the cancer.

Additional Resource

https://www.reviewofophthalmology.com/article/eyelid-lesions-diagnosis-and
   -treatment

Blepharospasm

LEON RAFAILOV, MD

What Is It? • Blepharospasm is a condition in which the muscles in the eyelids and around the eyes twitch uncontrollably. Both eyes are typically involved, and the spasms usually begin as mild twitches and can progress to forceful blinking. These symptoms are usually not present during sleep. The cause of most cases of blepharospasm is unknown. Older patients tend to be affected most often, and women are slightly more prone to the disorder than men. Severe blepharospasm can limit a person's ability to read, drive, or perform other daily activities. Sometimes, blepharospasm may be associated with spasm of other facial muscles. This condition, known as hemifacial spasm, can be due to compression of the facial nerve by a blood vessel and can occur even while sleeping.

Symptoms: What You May Experience • You may notice frequent, repeated twitching of your eyelids or forceful blinking of both eyes that you cannot control. It may be worse with bright lights, fatigue, or stress.

Examination Findings: What the Doctor Looks For • Your eye doctor will watch your eyelid movements to determine if blepharospasm is present. They may also check to see if other muscles of your face are involved. Your doctor will also look for any other causes of excessive blinking, such as dry eye syndrome. If you have hemifacial spasm, your doctor may order imaging to see if there is compression of the facial nerves.

What You Can Do • There is no proven way to avoid the development of blepharospasm. If blepharospasm is causing your eyes to feel irritated, a trial of artificial tear drops or lubricating ointment can help.

When to Call the Doctor • If you notice the symptoms of blepharospasm, call your eye doctor. Although blepharospasm itself is typically not dangerous, treating it can make you much more comfortable and allow you to function better in your daily activities.

Treatment • The main treatment for blepharospasm is an injection of botulinum toxin (often known by the brand name Botox, although other products exist) into the muscles around the eyes to partially paralyze them. In the office, your ophthalmologist will inject the botulinum toxin through the skin, using a tiny needle. The botulinum toxin will begin working in about 2–3 days, and it typically lasts for about 2–4 months, after which time the spasms usually reoccur and the botulinum toxin needs be injected again. The side effects of botulinum toxin are rare but include droopy eyelids, inability to fully close the eyelids, dry eye, and crossing or drifting of the eye(s). Your doctor may have to alter the pattern and dosage of the injections until they find a combination that works best for you.

Rarely, if botulinum toxin is not effective and the blepharospasm is severe, surgery can be considered. Your ophthalmologist will remove and weaken some of the surrounding eye muscles to reduce the blepharospasm permanently. You may still need botulinum toxin injections after surgery.

Prognosis: Will I See Better? • While blepharospasm is a longstanding disorder, most cases can be treated successfully with repeated botulinum toxin injections.

Additional Resource

https://eyewiki.aao.org/Blepharospasm

Conjunctivitis (Pink Eye)

S. GRACE PRAKALAPAKORN, MD, MPH

What Is It? • Conjunctivitis, or "pink eye," is a condition caused by inflammation of the thin layer of tissue (conjunctiva) that covers the inner surface of the eyelids and the front white surface of the eyeball (sclera). Conjunctivitis may be caused by many conditions including infections, most commonly bacterial and viral; non-infectious causes, in particular allergies including dust, pollen, animal dander, and medications; and other medical conditions such as immune-mediated diseases.

Symptoms: What You May Experience • The eye(s) can appear pink or red. There may be tearing or discharge and crusting of the eyelashes. Other symptoms include a burning, itching, or foreign body sensation. In cases of allergic conjunctivitis, itching is usually the major feature. In severe forms of conjunctivitis, you may also notice a decrease in vision.

Examination Findings: What the Doctor Looks For • The eye doctor will look for potential causes of the conjunctivitis. The conjunctiva will be examined to assess the severity of the disease and to look for signs that will help identify whether the conjunctivitis is caused by an infectious or non-infectious cause. The doctor will also look for involvement of the clear part of the eye (cornea), which can affect your vision. If there is severe purulent discharge draining from the eye(s), your doctor may send a sample of it to the laboratory to help identify the cause of the infection.

What You Can Do • If you have conjunctivitis due to a bacterial or viral infection, it is contagious. The most important thing that you can do is practice good hygiene. Hand washing is the best way to prevent the spread of infection. Avoid touching your eyes and do not share linens such as wash cloths, towels, pillows, or blankets to prevent the spread of the contagious forms of conjunctivitis to other people. In order to ensure your infection is fully treated, use any medications for the full length of time prescribed.

If you have allergic conjunctivitis, and you know the cause of your allergies, you can try to avoid or limit your contact with the allergens. Washing your face and using over-the-counter artificial tears can help decrease the amount of allergen that comes in contact with your eyes and reduce the allergic reaction. Also, try to avoid rubbing the eyes. The use of cold compresses can reduce the itching and swelling of the white of the eye and the eyelids. Allergic conjunctivitis can also be treated with allergy eye drops. If you have other allergy symptoms (for example a runny nose), you can also try using an oral allergy medication as suggested by your doctor.

When to Call the Doctor • It is important to seek medical care if any of the following symptoms are associated with the "pink eye": loss of vision, eye pain, severe discharge from the eye, failure to improve within 1–2 weeks, or worsening of symptoms.

Treatment • The treatment of conjunctivitis depends on the cause. Bacterial conjunctivitis may be treated with antibiotic drops or ointment. Viral conjunctivitis is not treated with antibiotics and usually resolves on its own over several weeks; however, you may be prescribed an antiviral medication in certain situations. Artificial tears and cool compresses may provide symptomatic relief. Allergic conjunctivitis can be treated with allergy eye drops. If the conjunctivitis is caused by a medication, it should resolve after the medication has been stopped. If the conjunctivitis is caused by another medical condition, treating the underlying medical condition may help the conjunctivitis.

Prognosis: Will I See Better? • In uncomplicated or mild cases of conjunctivitis, vision should not be affected. In more severe or complicated forms of conjunctivitis, vision may be affected from the associated tearing or discharge or involvement of the cornea. As the tearing and discharge decreases, your vision should improve. If there is involvement of the cornea, vision may be improved with the use of a treatment plan prescribed by your eye doctor.

Additional Resources

http://eyewiki.org/Conjunctivitis

https://www.aao.org/eye-health/diseases/pink-eye-conjunctivitis

Subconjunctival Hemorrhage

S. GRACE PRAKALAPAKORN, MD, MPH

What Is It? • A subconjunctival hemorrhage is an accumulation of blood in the space between the conjunctiva (the thin layer of tissue that covers the eyeball and inner surfaces of the eyelids) and the sclera (the white outer layer of the eyeball). A subconjunctival hemorrhage is commonly caused by a sudden increase in ocular venous pressure, which occurs with coughing, sneezing, vomiting, or rubbing the eye. They can also be caused by highly elevated blood pressure. Most subconjunctival hemorrhages occur in normal, healthy people. People who have bleeding disorders or take blood-thinning medications such as aspirin or warfarin may be more prone to having a subconjunctival hemorrhage.

Symptoms: What You May Experience • It is common to suddenly notice a bright red area over the normally white part of the eyeball. Occasionally, the red spot will look thickened and raised. A subconjunctival hemorrhage may cause a feeling of mild eye irritation but should not cause severe eye pain. Your vision is normally not affected. Often, a subconjunctival hemorrhage occurs during sleep or after coughing, sneezing, vomiting, or rubbing the eye. Most occur spontaneously and will resolve on their own over 1–2 weeks. Because the space between the conjunctiva and sclera encircles the colored part of the eye, it is not uncommon to see the hemorrhage spread or move to other parts of the white part of the eye while it is healing. You may also notice the hemorrhage change in color from red to yellow to green as it resolves.

Examination Findings: What the Doctor Looks For • The eye doctor will look for potential causes of the subconjunctival hemorrhage and ask if there has been any trauma to the eye. It is important to let your doctor know when you noticed the subconjunctival hemorrhage (for example, after straining or rubbing the eye or after an eye injury), if you bruise easily, tend to have bloody noses, if you take any medications that thin your blood (for example, aspirin or warfarin), or have high blood pressure, diabetes, or a bleeding disorder.

What You Can Do • To speed up the resolution of the hemorrhage, avoid taking any optional blood-thinning medications, such as nonsteroidal anti-inflammatory medications such as ibuprofen or aspirin, and avoid any trauma to the eye including rubbing the eyes. Don't stop blood thinners if you are taking them for a medical condition. If your eye feels irritated, you can use over-the-counter artificial tears to help relieve the irritation.

When to Call the Doctor • A subconjunctival hemorrhage has a striking appearance. Usually there is no danger of visual loss, but immediate medical attention should be sought if the subconjunctival hemorrhage developed after trauma to the eye. Seek medical attention if you have had a recurrent subconjunctival hemorrhage in order to be evaluated for a bleeding disorder or other systemic diseases.

Treatment • If the subconjunctival hemorrhage was not caused by trauma to the eye, treatment is not needed. Avoid taking any optional blood-thinning medications, such as ibuprofen, naproxen, or aspirin to speed up the resolution of the hemorrhage. If the eye feels irritated, you can use over-the-counter artificial tears to help with the irritation. If you have recurrent subconjunctival hemorrhage, you should be evaluated by a doctor to test for a possible bleeding disorder or other systemic disease.

Prognosis: Will I See Better? • In most cases, a subconjunctival hemorrhage will not affect your vision and will resolve in 1–2 weeks.

Additional Resource

https://www.aao.org/eye-health/diseases/what-is-subconjunctival-hemorrhage

Pingueculum and Pterygium (Surfer's Eye)

KRISTEN M. PETERSON, MD

What Is It? • A pingueculum is a growth, typically yellow and triangular, that develops on the layer of tissue, called the conjunctiva, that covers the inner surface of the eyelids and the front white surface of the eyeball. Pinguecula are composed of either protein, calcium, or fat and most commonly appear on the nasal side of the eye. A pterygium is a fleshy wedge-shaped growth over the conjunctiva that can extend onto the clear, round center part of the eye called the cornea. They typically grow on the nasal side of the white of the eyeball but can also grow on the part of the conjunctiva closer to the ear, or grow on both sides simultaneously.

Symptoms: What You May Experience • You may experience a gritty sensation in your eyes, eye redness, dryness, itching, or blurry vision. If large, a pterygium may cause your glasses prescription to change or interfere with the fit of your contact lenses.

Examination Findings: What the Doctor Looks For • Your eye doctor will use a slit lamp to examine the conjunctiva and cornea. They will look for signs of redness or inflammation at the site of the pingueculum or pterygium and will measure how far onto your cornea the pterygium extends. A special image of the cornea may be obtained to look for irregular astigmatism induced by the pterygium.

What You Can Do • Avoid ultraviolet light or sun exposure, dust, and wind by wearing sunglasses when outside. If a pingueculum or pterygium is causing your eyes to be red or irritated, using artificial tear drops and or lubricating eye ointment may be helpful.

When to Call the Doctor • If you have multiple episodes of eye redness or irritation at the site of a pingueculum or pterygium, call your eye doctor. If you have a known pterygium and you notice a decrease in vision, schedule an appointment with your eye doctor right away.

Treatment • While having a pingueculum or pterygium is not dangerous and these are noncancerous growths, surgical removal may be considered to alleviate recurrent episodes of redness, irritation, or if the pterygium begins to cause a decrease in vision.

Prognosis: Will I See Better? • Small pinguecula and small stationary pterygia can often be monitored. If surgical excision is recommended, pinguecula and pterygia can be removed from the surface of the eyeball to help restore the eye's appearance, treat symptoms of irritation, and improve vision that worsened as a result of the resulting astigmatism. Recurrence of the growth can occur, but precautions are taken at the time of surgery to decrease that risk.

Additional Resource

https://www.aao.org/eye-health/diseases/pinguecula-pterygium

Episcleritis

PRITHVI MRUTHYUNJAYA, MD, MHS

What Is It? • The episclera is the connective tissue layer underneath the conjunctiva that overlies the white part of the eye (sclera). The small fibers in the episclera can become inflamed, a condition termed episcleritis. The majority of cases are not caused by any systemic disease or eye infection.

Symptoms: What You May Experience • Episcleritis often causes painless irritation, tearing, redness, and itching of the eye. It rarely causes severe eye pain, discharge, or decreased vision.

Examination Findings: What the Doctor Looks For • Using the slit lamp, your eye doctor can identify episcleral inflammation while ruling out infection, glaucoma, or inflammation inside the eyeball (uveitis). Your eye doctor may confirm the diagnosis of episcleritis by using a certain dilating eye drop. The redness is typically localized in one sector of the eye surface and is not usually diffuse.

What You Can Do • There is no way to prevent the development of episcleritis.

When to Call the Doctor • If you notice eye redness that is associated with discharge, eye pain, or decreased vision, call your eye doctor promptly. Persistent eye redness by itself, without other symptoms, may be examined more routinely.

Treatment • Episcleritis usually resolves within a week, even without treatment. For comfort, artificial tears may be used. Medicated eye drops designed to reduce eye redness should be avoided, as they can worsen the condition in the long run. In severe cases, a steroid eye drop may be prescribed for a short time to control the inflammation. Oral anti-inflammatory medicines such as ibuprofen may also be prescribed in recurrent cases.

Prognosis: Will I See Better? • Although episcleritis usually resolves quickly without permanent consequences, you may experience repeated episodes. It is important to inform your eye doctor if your symptoms are recurrent, as additional laboratory or other testing may be indicated.

Additional Resource

https://eyewiki.aao.org/Episcleritis

Scleritis

PRITHVI MRUTHYUNJAYA, MD, MHS

What Is It? • Scleritis is inflammation of the sclera, the white, outer covering of the eyeball. This rare condition can affect either the front (anterior scleritis) or, more commonly, the back (posterior scleritis) of the eye. Scleritis differs from other causes of a red eye because of its possible association with infections as well as systemic diseases such as rheumatoid arthritis and systemic lupus erythematosus.

Symptoms: What You May Experience • Scleritis often causes severe eye pain and, sometimes, decreased vision. In anterior scleritis, the normally white part of the eyeball is typically red, either in a small area or larger area. Sometimes the areas of redness may have a gray-blue appearance due to overlying thinning of the white sclera due to inflammation. In posterior scleritis, vision may be severely decreased while the front of the eye may show little or no redness.

Examination Findings: What the Doctor Looks For • Anterior scleritis is diagnosed by examination with a slit lamp. The pattern of redness helps to classify the scleritis, while thinning of the sclera or cornea indicates more severe disease. Your eye doctor may dilate your pupils to look for posterior scleritis or other inflammation in the back of the eye. In posterior scleritis, ultrasound testing, fluorescein angiography (a photographic dye test), or a computed tomography (CT) scan can sometimes aid in making the diagnosis. Your eye doctor may order blood tests to determine if the scleritis is related to underlying systemic inflammation or infection and may recommend an evaluation by your primary care doctor.

What You Can Do • There is no proven way to prevent the development of scleritis.

When to Call the Doctor • If you notice eye redness that is associated with discharge, eye pain, or decreased vision, call your eye doctor promptly. You may be referred to an eye doctor who specializes in uveitis.

Treatment • Oral nonsteroidal anti-inflammatory drugs, such as indomethacin and ibuprofen, are the first line of treatment for scleritis. Steroid eye drops may be prescribed in some cases as well. In more severe cases, oral steroids and other systemic immunosuppressive medicines such as high dose steroid therapy, cyclosporine, or methotrexate may be used. Newer generation immunomodulatory drugs may also be used. Complications from scleritis such as thinning of the eye wall, retinal detachment, or perforation (break in the eye wall due to weakening from the scleritis) may require emergency eye surgery.

Prognosis: Will I See Better? • In cases of mild to moderate scleritis, you can maintain or recover excellent vision. In more severe cases, the type of scleritis, how long the inflammation lasts, and complications from either the disease or treatment will determine the extent of improvement. Followup visits with your primary care medical doctor are essential for any associated systemic illness.

Additional Resources

https://www.aao.org/eye-health/diseases/what-is-scleritis
https://eyewiki.aao.org/Scleritis

Dry Eye Syndrome

JULIA SONG, MD

What Is It? • Dry eye syndrome is an extremely common condition in which the tear film that lubricates the surface of the eye is abnormal. It is usually due to either decreased tear production or increased tear evaporation. Common causes of decreased tear production include Sjögren syndrome, which is an autoimmune disorder in which the lacrimal gland is dysfunctional; lacrimal gland disease; and decreased corneal sensation. Common causes of excessive tear evaporation include blepharitis in which the oil glands around the eyelashes are clogged, blink problems, and eyelid-closing problems. Other causes of dry eye syndrome include systemic diseases such as sarcoidosis; certain medications such as antihistamines, decongestants, blood pressure medications, and antipsychotic agents; glaucoma eye drops; and prolonged wearing of contact lenses. Postmenopausal women may be especially prone to developing dry eye syndrome. Most cases of dry eye syndrome are not associated with a general medical disease or serious eye problem.

Symptoms: What You May Experience • You may experience a burning sensation in the eye(s), dryness, the feeling that something is in the eye, blurry vision, and sensitivity to light. These symptoms are often worse at the end of the day, or during times when you blink less such as while watching TV, reading, or spending time on the computer.

Examination Findings: What the Doctor Looks For • The eye doctor may see redness or swelling on the white of the eye, decreased tear film, debris in the tear film, an irregular surface of the cornea, or a poor blink response. The doctor may put an eye drop in your eye to check for certain staining patterns on your cornea or conjunctiva. In more severe cases, the doctor may find filaments and mucous plaques, which can be quite painful. In extremely severe cases, your cornea can become thin or, rarely, even perforate.

What You Can Do • You can reduce your chances of dry eye by avoiding medications that can cause dry eye, such as antihistamines and decongestants, and by decreasing the amount of time you wear contact lenses.

When to Call the Doctor • If you are experiencing persistent burning and dryness or any decrease in vision, redness, severe pain, or a white spot on the normally clear front surface of your eye, you should contact your eye doctor immediately. Certain causes of dry eye can lead to an increased risk of corneal infections.

Treatment • For mild dry eyes, treatment consists of over-the-counter, preservative-free artificial tear drops, administered up to four times a day, and lubricating ointment at night. There are prescription lubricating eyedrops, such as the brands Restasis (cyclosporine 0.05%) and Xiidra (lifitegrast). The newest medication is Cequa (cyclosporine 0.09%). These prescription lubricating eye drops are preservative-free, which means they do not have the preservative benzalkonium chloride, which can sometimes worsen dry eyes. If your eyes are moderately dry, you can use the preservative-free over-the-counter artificial tear drops more frequently, up to every hour if needed, as well as an ointment at night.

Artificial tears can range in viscosity. The thinner drops (Refresh Plus, for example) are more watery; they work well but only last 3–4 minutes. The thicker drops (such as Refresh Celluvisc or Systane Ultra preservative-free) last longer. There are many options in the store to choose from. Thicker drops can be more effective; however, they can cause temporarily blurred vision because they are gooey and sticky. These thicker drops form a hard crust on the eyelashes. The stickiness allows allergens and other chemicals to stick to the tear film. So, there is a tradeoff.

Another eye drop option is autologous serum, otherwise known as blood tears. It is made from your own serum. Several tubes of your blood are spun down with a centrifuge machine by your doctor or a laboratory. The cells are removed, and the top liquid part (serum) is saved. It contains many important growth factors and nutrients normally found in healthy tears. The serum can be diluted with a sterile, preservative-free solution to adjust the concentration. Because they are not preserved, store the drops in the freezer until you need them. They may not be covered by insurance.

If you do not want to use eye drops or ointment, your eye doctor may place plugs in your tear ducts so that tears will last longer in your eyes.

Collagen plugs are temporary as they melt away after 2 weeks. Permanent methods include plastic (silicone) plugs or punctal cautery, in which the tear ducts are cauterized closed. This can be performed in the office.

Another method to treat dry eyes is Lacrisert, a small (5 mg), sterile, clear insert that is water-soluble and preservative-free. The insert is placed into the inferior pocket (cul-de-sac) inside the lower eyelid once daily instead of using eye drops multiple times a day. It can cause temporary blurred vision.

LipiFlow is an electronic device approved by the Food and Drug Administration (FDA) to treat dry eye. With specialized goggles, heat is applied to the inner eyelids with directed gentle massage to remove blockages from the meibomian glands to restore the natural oil flow to the tear film that covers the eye's surface to prevent evaporation of your tear film. It is a 12-minute procedure. Results can be seen in 6–8 weeks. Intense pulsed light also can be used to treat dry eye. If your dry eye is due to blepharitis, then oral doxycycline (50 mg twice daily) can be considered. Other things that can help include a humidifier, fish oil, or flax seed.

Prognosis: Will I See Better? • Most patients maintain excellent vision with conservative management such as using artificial tears and lubricating ointment.

Additional Resources
https://www.aao.org/eye-health/diseases/what-is-dry-eye
https://eyewiki.aao.org/Dry_Eye_Syndrome

Infectious Keratitis

JULIA SONG, MD

What Is It? • Keratitis means inflammation of the cornea, the round clear central portion on the front of the eye. Causes include infection, dry eye syndrome, blepharitis, and autoimmune disorders. Infectious keratitis refers specifically to keratitis caused by a bacterial, viral, or fungal infection. A parasitic infection due to an amoeba called acanthamoeba can cause a severe and difficult-to-treat keratitis. Acanthamoeba infections are more commonly associated with contact lens wearers who wear the lenses while in the swimming pool or hot tub, or who wash their contact lenses in water. People who wear contact lenses are especially prone to infectious keratitis, and their risk of infection increases as they wear their contact lenses for longer periods. Infectious keratitis can develop into a corneal ulcer if the infection becomes severe.

Symptoms: What You May Experience • You may experience eye pain, redness, decreased vision, and sensitivity to light. The severity of your symptoms may depend on which type of bacterium, virus, or fungus is causing the infection.

Examination Findings: What the Doctor Looks For • The eye doctor looks for infection in the front of the eye with a slit lamp. Signs of infection include redness of the conjunctiva, whitening of the normally clear cornea, corneal swelling, abnormal new blood vessels growing in the cornea, and inflammatory cells in the cornea or front part of the eye. The eye doctor may scrape a sample from the surface of the cornea for laboratory evaluation to determine what type of bacterium, virus, fungus, or parasite is causing the infection.

What You Can Do • Avoid eye injury and keep dirt or foreign objects from entering your eyes. Wash your hands thoroughly before touching your eyes or handling contact lenses. Avoid sleeping in contact lenses.

When to Call the Doctor • If you are experiencing any decrease in vision, redness, severe pain, or a white spot on the normally clear front surface of your eye, you should call your eye doctor immediately. Avoid wearing contact lenses if you are having any such eye problem.

Treatment • Treatment depends on the underlying cause of the infectious keratitis. Appropriate antibiotic eye drops, such as antibacterial, antiviral, or antifungal agents, will likely be prescribed for frequent use (as often as every 30 to 60 minutes in severe infections). In certain cases, oral antibiotics can also help treat the infection.

Prognosis: Will I See Better? • Vision often improves with treatment of the underlying infection. However, there may be some scarring of the cornea after treatment that may or may not alter the vision in the long run. If the corneal scarring is in the center of the cornea, where it affects the line of sight, a corneal transplant may ultimately be needed to improve the vision.

Additional Resources
https://eyewiki.aao.org/Bacterial_Keratitis
https://eyewiki.aao.org/Fungal_Keratitis

Corneal Abrasion

JULIA SONG, MD

What Is It? • A corneal abrasion, also known as a corneal epithelial defect, is a scratch on the cornea, the clear central surface of the eye. An abrasion can be caused by an eye injury such as from a fingernail, a paper cut, a foreign body, or a contact lens.

Symptoms: What You May Experience • You may have immediate pain, the feeling that something is in your eye (gritty/sandy sensation), tearing, or discomfort with blinking. Corneal abrasions can be very painful because the cornea has many sensory nerves.

Examination Findings: What the Doctor Looks For • Your doctor may use an eye drop that has a special dye to see an area of staining where the top layer, or epithelium, of the cornea is missing. Your doctor may also see redness and inflammation of your eye.

What You Can Do • Avoid injury to your eyes and wear protective glasses when doing activities that put you at risk for debris getting into your eye such as yard work. Decrease the length of time you wear your contact lenses and be careful inserting and removing them.

When to Call the Doctor • If you are experiencing any decrease in vision, redness, severe pain, discharge, or a white spot on the normally clear central surface of your eye, you should contact your eye doctor immediately.

Treatment • Treatment usually depends on the size and cause of the abrasion. If it is small, it can be treated with antibiotic eye drops or ointment. If it is larger, antibiotic drops, certain dilating drops, a protective contact lens, and/or (rarely) pressure patching may be beneficial. If the abrasion is persistent, an amniotic membrane, which provides nutrients to the cornea, can be placed. If organic material (such as grass, plants, or wood) is the cause of the abrasion, then the abrasion is considered dirty and the eye will need to be examined more frequently for possible secondary infection. No pressure patching is recommended for abrasions caused by organic material or contact lenses.

Prognosis: Will I See Better? • Corneal abrasions generally heal in several days, with vision returning to normal. A secondary infection may make treatment more difficult and increases the chance of corneal scarring which can impact visual recovery. If you have diabetes, it may take longer for the corneal abrasion to heal.

Additional Resources

https://www.aao.org/eye-health/diseases/what-is-corneal-abrasion

https://eyewiki.aao.org/Corneal_Epithelial_Defect

Recurrent Corneal Erosion Syndrome

JULIA SONG, MD

What Is It? • This syndrome consists of recurrent corneal abrasions due to a loose top layer of the cornea called the epithelium. There may be a history of a corneal abrasion that occurred weeks, months, or years before the current episode. During the healing process, the corneal epithelium does not bind well to its underlying membrane and remains somewhat looser than normal, making future abrasions more likely. If you have a corneal epithelial basement membrane dystrophy, then you are at risk for developing recurrent corneal erosions spontaneously or with mild trauma. Other predisposing conditions include meibomian gland dysfunction (clogged oil glands around the eyelashes), diabetes, prior corneal infection, other corneal dystrophies, or refractive surgery such as LASIK.

Symptoms: What You May Experience • You may experience the feeling that something is in your eye, intense eye pain, or tearing. These symptoms often occur upon awakening.

Examination Findings: What the Doctor Looks For • Your eye doctor may use a yellow eye drop to see an area of green staining on the cornea using a blue light, where the epithelium of the cornea is missing. Your doctor may find that the top layer of the cornea looks rough and irregular. If the cause is a corneal epithelial basement membrane dystrophy, your doctor may see corneal abnormalities in your other eye.

What You Can Do • Avoid trauma if possible and minimize rubbing of the eye.

When to Call the Doctor • If you experience any decrease in vision, redness, severe pain, discharge, or a white spot on the front clear surface of your eye, you should contact your eye doctor immediately.

Treatment • Conservative management for acute recurrent erosions often consists of frequent lubrication with an antibiotic ointment. Hypertonic saline (5% sodium chloride) eye drops can also be used. In more severe cases, your eye doctor may prescribe a bandage contact lens. If there is associated inflammation, steroid eye drops may be added.

If conservative management does not work, anterior stromal puncture may be performed. In this technique, your eye doctor makes tiny puncture marks in the affected areas of the cornea with a needle, so that the top layer of the cornea will heal and stick more tightly to the underlying membrane. This is done in the clinic. Another treatment option is epithelial debridement, which involves peeling off the corneal epithelium. A bandage contact lens is used for several days afterward, until the epithelium regenerates. Phototherapeutic keratectomy, a laser procedure, has been found useful in rare cases.

Prognosis: Will I See Better? • Vision often returns to normal when the erosion has healed. A secondary infection may limit visual recovery. In some cases, there may be scarring of the cornea after treatment that may affect visual recovery, especially if scarring occurs in the center of the cornea.

Additional Resource
https://eyewiki.aao.org/Recurrent_Corneal_Erosion

Corneal Ulcer

ROSANNA P. BAHADUR, MD AND
NATALIE A. AFSHARI, MD

What Is It? • A corneal ulcer is a deep infection in the cornea (the clear front surface of the eye). The infection usually develops after an injury to the cornea, such as a corneal abrasion, and is often associated with wearing contact lenses. The type of organism causing the infection is usually a bacterium or fungus. Corneal ulcers can be very aggressive and harmful if not treated early by a qualified eye doctor, usually a cornea specialist.

Symptoms: What You May Experience • If you develop a corneal ulcer, you may notice a decrease in your vision, tearing, eye discharge, eye pain or redness, or sensitivity to light. When you look in the mirror, you may see a white spot on the normally clear cornea.

Examination Findings: What the Doctor Looks For • Your eye doctor will examine your cornea with a slit lamp to look for a scratch on the cornea and for any infection beneath it. Your doctor will also look for infection and inflammation in the tissues surrounding the cornea and inside the eye itself. If a corneal ulcer is large or located in the center of the cornea, your eye doctor may perform cultures to identify the specific bacteria or fungus causing the infection. The ulcer will be measured so that its size and progress can be followed from visit to visit.

What You Can Do • Use eye protection and avoid eye rubbing to prevent a corneal abrasion. If you think you may have scratched your eye, remove your contact lenses. Avoid sleeping in contact lenses, and never use tap water or saliva to clean your lenses.

When to Call the Doctor • If you think your eye may be scratched or if you develop vision loss, tearing, eye discharge, eye pain or redness, or sensitivity to light, call your eye doctor promptly. Be sure to mention any history of contact lens wear or trauma.

Treatment • Your eye doctor may prescribe antibiotic eye drops to target the bacteria or fungus causing the infection. These antibiotic eye drops may need to be used as often as every 30 minutes. Your doctor may also prescribe a dilating eye drop to decrease eye pain and later steroid drops to decrease inflammation. You will likely have frequent eye exams while the corneal ulcer is being treated (sometimes every day or every other day). If the ulcer causes significant corneal scarring after it has healed, a corneal transplant may ultimately be necessary in rare cases.

Prognosis: Will I See Better? • Many people have improved vision after a corneal ulcer has healed. In cases where scarring of the cornea occurs and affects the vision, the vision may be poor unless a corneal transplant is performed.

Additional Resources

https://www.aao.org/eye-health/diseases/corneal-ulcer

https://eyewiki.aao.org/Bacterial_Keratitis

Keratoconus

ROSANNA P. BAHADUR, MD AND NATALIE A. AFSHARI, MD

What Is It? • The cornea is the clear, dome-shaped surface that covers the front central area of the eyeball and focuses light onto the retina. In keratoconus, the cornea is abnormally shaped because the middle area is thin and bulges out, resulting in a cornea that is cone shaped rather than smoothly curved. Mild cases may cause distorted vision because of the cornea's shape. In moderate or severe keratoconus, the thinned cornea can develop tiny cracks that lead to corneal swelling and eye pain. Scarring of the cornea can also occur.

In the United States, keratoconus occurs in about 1 of every 2,000 people, most of whom are diagnosed in their teens or early twenties. The shape of the cornea in keratoconus tends to stabilize after young adulthood. When present, keratoconus is almost always found in both eyes, but one eye may be worse than the other. The cause of the disease is not known, but keratoconus can run in families and has been linked to frequent eye rubbing, long-term use of contact lenses, Down syndrome, and other rare diseases.

Symptoms: What You May Experience • You may have trouble seeing clearly, even with a new eyeglass prescription, and your prescription may change significantly over time, particularly between regular eye exams. If you wear contact lenses, the lenses may easily fall out of your eyes.

Examination Findings: What the Doctor Looks For • The eye doctor will examine the shape of your cornea with a slit lamp and look for thin or steep areas. Specialized photographs of the cornea, called corneal topography, may be taken to measure the cornea's steepness and shape.

What You Can Do • Reduce the number of hours you wear contact lenses and avoid rubbing your eyes excessively. Keeping up with regular eye exams can help your eye doctor notice if your glasses prescription changes rapidly.

When to Call the Doctor • If you notice decreased vision despite a new eyeglass prescription, you should call your eye doctor. If you have keratoconus and experience eye pain, excessive tearing, or decreased vision, call your eye doctor, since these symptoms could mean that your cornea has thinned to a certain point and needs treatment.

Treatment • In mild keratoconus, properly prescribed eyeglasses or, more commonly, hard contact lenses usually improve vision by compensating for the steepness of the cornea. Episodes of sudden corneal swelling may be treated with eye drops or a soft contact lens. A newly approved office technique to strengthen corneal tissue, called corneal crosslinking, may be an option for milder cases. In moderate or severe keratoconus, a corneal transplant may ultimately be needed.

Prognosis: Will I See Better? • Most keratoconus patients do very well with hard contact lenses. If corneal transplantation is necessary, these patients tend to heal well, and many experience good vision afterward.

Additional Resources
https://www.nkcf.org/understanding-kc/
https://eyewiki.aao.org/Keratoconus

Fuchs Endothelial Corneal Dystrophy

BRENTON D. FINKLEA, MD

What Is It? • Fuchs endothelial corneal dystrophy is a genetic condition caused by abnormal cells of the inner layer of the cornea (corneal endothelium). The disease usually begins to manifest symptoms after the age of 50. As the disease progresses, the unhealthy endothelial cells cause edema (swelling) of the normally clear cornea, which can impair vision. This is a relatively common condition, found in nearly 4% of the population when examined by their eye doctor. Because Fuchs has a broad spectrum of severity, only a fraction of affected individuals require medical or surgical therapy for improvement of their vision.

Symptoms: What You May Experience • Early stages have no symptoms or discomfort and vision remains clear. As Fuchs progresses, you may experience progressive blurring of your vision, halos around lights, and hazy vision. Often the blurry or hazy vision is worse in the morning and improves throughout the day. Irritation may occur as a result of the cornea swelling. Sudden sharp pain or a foreign body sensation in the eye may be due to abrasions on the surface as a result of advanced swelling. Light sensitivity may accompany these periods of pain.

Exam Findings: What the Doctor Looks For
Before any visual changes occur, your eye doctor will closely examine the back surface of the cornea for guttata—the visible effects of an unhealthy corneal endothelium. Your eye doctor will see small bumps on the back surface of your cornea. In the later stages, corneal edema will cause the normally clear cornea to become slightly opaque, hazy, and thickened.

What You Can Do • Due to the genetic nature of Fuchs, there is currently no way to cure it without surgery to remove the malfunctioning corneal cells. Early visual manifestations of Fuchs can be treated by carefully and appropriately pointing a blow dryer toward your eyes and face in the morning to help evaporate excess fluid and moisture (edema), which has collected overnight in your cornea. Artificial tears may be used to soothe irritation. Regular ophthalmic exams to monitor the Fuchs are necessary to determine what treatments may be helpful and if surgery may be necessary.

When to Call the Doctor • Pain is uncommon in Fuchs dystrophy except in the most advanced cases with significant corneal edema. Worsening of haze, fog, or blurring of your vision may indicate that the Fuchs is progressing. Schedule a routine visit with your eye doctor if you experience these progressive symptoms to evaluate the status of the disease. If you develop sudden pain, light sensitivity, eye redness or severe worsening of your vision, contact your physician promptly. Scratches or abrasions may form on the cornea as a result of significant swelling, and in rare cases, these may become infected.

Treatment • Treatment becomes necessary when the vision is affected by corneal edema or light scatter from the unhealthy endothelium. Hypertonic sodium chloride drops may be used to clear the cornea when mild amounts of edema are present. If the edema worsens, then surgery may be necessary. Descemet stripping endothelial keratoplasty (DSEK) or Descemet membrane endothelial keratoplasty (DMEK) are forms of partial-thickness corneal transplantation used to replace the unhealthy endothelium with a healthy piece of tissue from a deceased donor.

Prognosis • Fuchs endothelial corneal dystrophy has a very good prognosis, as it often progresses very slowly and has multiple treatment options at various stages of the disease. Close management by your eye doctor is key to a positive long-term visual outcome.

Additional Resource
https://eyewiki.aao.org/Fuchs'_Endothelial_Dystrophy

Corneal Transplantation

ROSANNA P. BAHADUR, MD AND NATALIE A. AFSHARI, MD

Why Is Corneal Transplantation Performed? • When a normally clear cornea becomes cloudy, it blocks light from reaching the retina, resulting in decreased vision. If this happens to you, your eye doctor may decide that a corneal transplant is needed to improve your vision. A corneal transplant is a surgery in which a diseased cornea is replaced with a clear, healthy, donor cornea. Sometimes the entire full thickness cornea is replaced, while in other cases, just part of the cornea is replaced, such as the innermost layer called the endothelium.

Where Do Donor Corneas Come From? • Donor corneas come from people who have agreed to donate their eye tissue after they die to help others regain their sight. After a donor dies, the corneas are removed and taken to an eye bank, where they are examined to make sure they are healthy. The cornea is unique, because, unlike other transplanted organs, it does not have to be immunologically matched to the patient receiving the transplant. The eye bank keeps the donor corneas until they are needed for corneal transplant surgery.

What Happens during Corneal Transplant Surgery? • Corneal transplantation is an outpatient surgery performed in the operating room. You are given intravenous sedation and numbing medicine is placed around the eye so that the operation is painless. The diseased cornea is removed us-

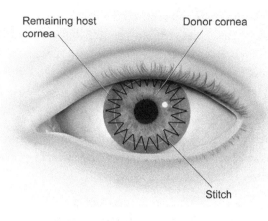

7.1. Corneal transplant.

ing an instrument called a trephine that resembles a cookie cutter. Next, a healthy donor cornea is cut to fit and then sutured into place with microscopic sutures. When a partial corneal transplant is done, sometimes sutures aren't needed, but instead an air or gas bubble is used to keep the partially transplanted cornea in the right place. This procedure usually takes 60–90 minutes and is followed by a short recovery time.

What Should I Expect after Corneal Transplant Surgery? • After surgery, your cornea surgeon will check your eye the next day. Your surgeon will prescribe antibiotic and steroid eye drops to be used while the transplant heals. Normal activities can be resumed after corneal transplantation, with some limitations. Heavy lifting, bending, or straining should be avoided after surgery until approved by your surgeon. Some form of eye protection should be worn at all times after surgery. It is normal to feel scratchiness and eye irritation for some time after the surgery.

Will My Vision Improve after Corneal Transplantation? • The improvement in vision after a corneal transplant is different for each patient, but achieving the best possible vision usually takes 6 to 12 months. At each follow-up exam, your cornea surgeon may remove some of the stitches, if present, which is a painless procedure performed in the office, to reduce visual distortion caused by astigmatism. You may achieve your best vision after a corneal transplant by wearing a hard contact lens. You will likely need to use a steroid eye drop long term to help prevent your body from rejecting the transplanted cornea and causing it to fail.

As with all surgeries, there are risks and benefits of corneal transplantation, such as infection and bleeding among others; your eye doctor will discuss these with you. After surgery, using the recommended eye drops and keeping your scheduled follow-up exams will give your new cornea the best chance to improve your vision.

Additional Resources

https://eyewiki.aao.org/Penetrating_Keratoplasty
https://restoresight.org/
http://www.nlm.nih.gov/medlineplus/ency/article/003008.htm

Cataract

TERRY SEMCHYSHYN, MD

What Is It? • A cataract is a natural clouding of the normally clear lens inside the eye that can make the vision hazy. The lens sits in the eye, just behind the iris and pupil. Light must pass through the lens to reach the retina. Cataracts are part of the natural aging process and are found in over 75% of people over the age of 70. The lens is clear at birth, but with time, it becomes hazier and more yellow or brown.

Cataracts are one of the most common causes of treatable, reversible vision loss. The most common type of cataract is an age-related cataract. Much less commonly, cataracts can be present at birth; these are called congenital cataracts. A cataract that forms as a result of an eye injury is a traumatic cataract. Certain medical conditions (such as diabetes) and certain medicines (such as steroids) can cause cataracts to become cloudy at a faster rate. However, it is impossible to predict how quickly a cataract will progress. In most cases, cataracts do not cause permanent damage to the eye but they do affect the vision until they are treated. However, very rare cases of extremely advanced cataracts may result in inflammation or high eye pressure.

Symptoms: What You May Experience • Your vision may gradually become blurry over months or years, and you may notice sensitivity to light or glare (starbursts or halos around lights). Poor night vision, difficulty driving, and need for brighter lighting are common symptoms of cataracts. Some people also experience double vision in one eye, fading or yellowing of colors, or frequent eyeglass prescription changes, especially after years of stable vision. Cataracts may cause some people to no longer need their eyeglasses as the cataract changes the way the eye refracts, or bends, light (known as "second sight"). Cataracts are typically painless.

Cataracts—the word means "waterfall"—are so named because having a cataract may give the impression of looking through mist or fog from a waterfall.

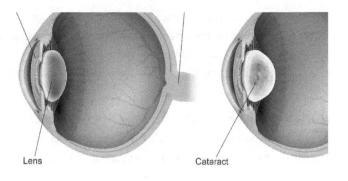

Lens   Cataract

8.1. Left: normal lens. Right: cataract lens.

Examination Findings: What the Doctor Looks For • Your eye doctor will notice that your vision may be blurred, even with the best glasses prescription. Your doctor may also perform a "glare test" by shining bright lights toward your eyes while you read the eye chart. This test simulates glare from sunshine or car headlights. Your doctor may dilate your pupils to see the lens better and will also look for other possible causes of your blurry vision.

What You Can Do • There are no known medicines, vitamin supplements, or exercises that can prevent or cure cataracts. Wearing sunglasses as protection from excess ultraviolet (UV) light may help slow the progression of cataracts.

When to Call the Doctor • Call your doctor if you start to notice painless blurry vision, glare, sensitivity to light, or poor vision in dim light. Cataracts do not harm the eye in most cases, but they do cause your vision to become blurrier over time. Trouble with driving, especially at night, and having to use brighter lights to read comfortably are other reasons to call your eye doctor. Sometimes the blurry vision is not due to cataracts but to another eye condition; that is why it is important to call your eye doctor if you notice any changes in your vision.

Treatment • Cataract surgery should be considered when the cataract causes enough blurriness to interfere with your daily activities. Surgery is the only known way to treat cataracts. It can improve vision and make colors seem brighter. If a cataract makes your vision only slightly blurry and is not bothersome, then a follow-up visit in several months or a year may be recommended before it is decided whether cataract surgery is needed.

Prognosis: Will I See Better? • Cataract surgery is one of the most common and most successful surgeries performed in the United States today. If a cataract is the main cause of blurry vision, then your chance of seeing better after cataract surgery is quite good.

Additional Resources

https://eyewiki.aao.org/Cataract

https://www.aao.org/eye-health/diseases/what-are-cataracts

https://nei.nih.gov/learn-about-eye-health/eye-conditions-and-diseases/cataracts

Cataract Surgery

TERRY SEMCHYSHYN, MD

What Is It? • Once your eye doctor has diagnosed a cataract that is affecting your vision, using surgery to remove the cloudy lens is the only way to treat it. In small-incision surgery, a tiny opening (1/8 of an inch) is made in the eye, then a special instrument that uses ultrasound energy breaks the cataract into small pieces and removes them—this process is called phacoemulsification. A permanent, clear, artificial lens implant is then inserted inside the eye in place of the natural lens to help focus light. A stitch may or may not be used to close the small opening in the eye at the end of the operation. Your eye surgeon performs this extremely delicate surgery with a powerful magnifying microscope. There are different lens implants available, some of which may also help improve distance and near vision as well as astigmatism. It may also be performed with the assistance of a laser, but this is not essential.

What You May Experience • Once you and your doctor have decided to proceed with cataract surgery, your eye will be measured in the office for the new artificial lens implant. Your surgery will usually be an outpatient or same-day surgery, meaning that you will come to the hospital the day of the surgery and go home after the operation on the same day.

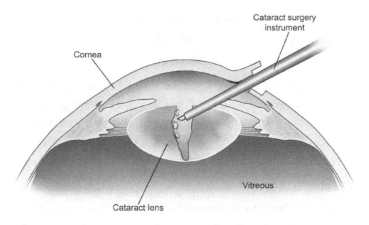

Cataract surgery instrument

Cornea

Vitreous

Cataract lens

8.2. Instrument placed in eyeball for cataract surgery.

You will be asked not to eat or drink after midnight the night before your surgery to avoid having an upset stomach during your surgery.

Most patients are not put completely to sleep (general anesthesia) for cataract surgery, but instead may be given intravenous sedation to relax as well as numbing eye drops or a numbing injection around the eye. During the surgery, you may hear your surgeon speak or the sound of instruments working, and you may see bright lights and changing colors, but you will not see the details of the actual surgery. Near the end of your surgery, the microscope light may become very bright as your lens implant is fitted inside your eye. Sometimes a dissolvable stitch is placed. Once the surgery is over, your doctor may put a small shield over your eye to protect it.

After visiting the recovery area and having something to eat or drink, you are usually able to go home. You may be asked to use eye drops after your surgery. Your eye doctor will usually see you in the office the next morning and several times afterward. You will likely need a new glasses prescription several weeks after surgery. If you have cataracts in both eyes, only one eye is treated at a time; usually the second cataract can be removed several weeks to several months after the first.

Examination Findings: What the Doctor Looks for • During your eye exams after cataract surgery, your eye doctor checks for inflammation, infection, and proper position of the lens implant. Most patients do not experience any significant pain or discomfort, and pain medication is not typically needed.

What You Can Do • Make sure you take all medicines and eye drops as directed. After surgery, your doctor may ask you to wear glasses during the day and an eye shield while sleeping to protect your eye. Avoid dusty or dirty areas, and do not bend over at the waist. Ask your doctor when you can return to driving (often as soon as the next afternoon) and your usual physical activity.

When to Call the Doctor • While cataract surgery usually goes very well, every surgery has risks of complications. Possible complications of cataract surgery include bleeding, infection, needing further surgery, a poor cosmetic result, retinal detachment, high eye pressure, and, extremely rarely, even loss of vision or of the eye itself. After surgery, you should call your eye doctor immediately if your vision worsens, if you have eye pain, if you vomit, if you injure your eye, or if anything seems worse.

Prognosis: Will I See Better? • Cataract surgery is one of the more successful surgeries performed today, and visual improvement is often excellent. Sometimes other eye problems, such as glaucoma, diabetic retinopathy, or macular degeneration, can limit your potential vision. However, even with such limits, cataract surgery may still help make your vision brighter or improve your side vision.

Additional Resources

https://www.aao.org/eye-health/diseases/what-is-cataract-surgery
https://eyewiki.aao.org/Cataract

Posterior Capsule Opacification ("After Cataract")

TERRY SEMCHYSHYN, MD

What Is It? • Following cataract surgery, a thin film or haze, called a posterior capsular opacity or "after cataract," can form behind the lens implant in some eyes. This film is caused by remaining microscopic lens cells that continue to grow on the naturally clear capsule that holds the intraocular lens implant in place. Usually this haze develops a few months after cataract surgery but it can be present sooner. It is painless and harmless to the eye but causes the vision to become more blurred over time.

Symptoms: What You May Experience • Your vision may slowly become blurry over the months following cataract surgery. You may notice glare with bright lights at night, and in fact, you may have changes in your vision similar to those that you experienced while you still had your original cataract.

Examination Findings: What the Doctor Looks For • Your eye doctor may be able to detect a posterior capsular opacity during your visits after surgery by examining your eye. Your doctor will see a hazy film on the capsule behind your lens implant. If your eye doctor thinks the film is thick enough to affect your vision, they may recommend laser treatment.

What You Can Do • There is no way for you to prevent a posterior capsular opacity from forming. A new glasses prescription will not improve vision because the light must still travel through the haze to get to the retina of the eye.

When to Call the Doctor • You should call your eye doctor if you notice your vision getting hazier and blurrier after cataract surgery. If you have recently had the laser treatment and you notice flashing lights, many new floaters, or a dark curtain anywhere in your vision, call your surgeon immediately. These changes could be warning signs of a retinal detachment that would need urgent treatment.

Treatment • About 50% of the eyes that develop a posterior capsular opacity will need a laser treatment to improve the vision. The laser treatment is usually done in your surgeon's office and does not require a visit to the operating room. Your eye doctor may use a special contact lens on your eye to help guide the laser. The treatment itself normally takes several minutes. The laser makes an opening in this haze on the posterior capsule so light can travel clearly into your eye. The opening is sized to fit your pupil. Afterward, your eye doctor may check your eye pressure and ask you to use steroid eye drops for a few days to suppress any inflammation from the laser procedure. In general, laser treatment for a posterior capsular opacity is low risk. However, rare complications from the laser include high eye pressure, inflammation, retinal detachment, and dislocation of the lens implant.

Prognosis: Will I See Better? • Posterior capsular opacities can generally be removed with laser surgery, often improving vision. After this haze is treated by laser, it does not grow back.

Additional Resources

https://www.aao.org/eye-health/treatments/what-is-posterior-capsulotomy

https://eyewiki.aao.org/Posterior_capsule_opacification

Dislocated Lens

TERRY SEMCHYSHYN, MD

What Is It? • Dislocation of either a natural lens or a lens implant after cataract surgery means that the lens has shifted from its proper position within the eye. If the shift is large enough, it can cause blurry vision, similar to how the vision might change if your glasses slid down to the tip of your nose. Dislocation of a natural lens can happen after eye injury or spontaneously because of certain medical conditions.

Dislocation of a lens implant after cataract surgery can also occur. During cataract surgery, a permanent artificial lens implant is often placed in the eye to improve vision. The lens implant is usually supported by the same capsular bag that gave support to the original natural lens. This bag normally supports the lens implant adequately, but it can shift or develop openings that can cause the lens implant that is supported by it to shift.

A lens or lens implant that shifts but stays within the capsular bag is called a subluxed lens. A dislocated lens, on the other hand, occurs if the lens or lens implant moves out of the bag, or if both the bag and the lens move away from their normal positions. Both subluxation and dislocation of a lens or lens implant can cause blurry vision.

Symptoms: What You May Experience • You may experience blurry vision or double vision, both of which may worsen over time. Wearing glasses does not usually improve the vision.

What the Doctor Looks For • Your eye doctor will check the position of your lens or lens implant using a slit lamp microscope.

What You Can Do • The only way you can sometimes prevent lens dislocation is to avoid eye injury. Follow your doctor's instructions about eye protection after cataract surgery.

When to Call the Doctor • Call your eye doctor if you have double vision that is not improved by your glasses or if your vision suddenly becomes worse.

Treatment • A lens or lens implant that is only slightly out of position may not affect your vision enough to need treatment or it may be in a location that does not require its removal. A subluxed or dislocated natural lens may need to be removed with surgery. A subluxed or dislocated lens implant may be put back in its proper location with surgery or possibly exchanged with a lens implant that can be anchored differently to the eye.

Prognosis: Will I See Better? • Often surgery for lens subluxation or dislocation is quite successful in improving vision. Rarely, the dislocated lens or lens implant may damage the retina or other important parts inside the eye, ultimately limiting your vision.

Additional Resources

https://eyewiki.aao.org/Ectopia_Lentis

https://www.asrs.org/patients/retinal-diseases/27/intraocular-lens-dislocation

9 · Age-Related Macular Degeneration

ANKUR MEHRA, MD AND RAMIRO S. MALDONADO, MD

What Is It? • Age-related macular degeneration (AMD) is a common degenerative disorder of the retina. AMD affects the macula, which is the part of the retina responsible for central vision and allows you to read, drive, look at a computer or phone screen, and see faces. The exact cause of AMD is not known, but it is closely associated with aging, which is the biggest risk factor. Genetic and hereditary factors, such as family history and ethnicity, also play a role. While these factors cannot be changed, others can be. Stopping smoking and reducing cholesterol, high blood pressure, and UV light exposure can all lower your risk.

AMD is typically classified into two groups: non-exudative, which is often called "dry" AMD, and exudative, or "wet" AMD. In dry AMD, collections of cellular waste products, called drusen, develop underneath the retina. Over time, drusen can be associated with cell damage in the central retina, resulting in slow progressive vision loss. Dry AMD is graded as early, intermediate, or advanced based on the number and size of drusen, as well as whether or not there is atrophy of the supporting cells underlying the retina, called the retinal pigment epitheliu (RPE). Sometimes, dry AMD converts into wet AMD, which is less common but can progress much more quickly. Wet AMD is characterized by the growth of abnormal new blood vessels underneath the retina, called choroidal neovascularization, and can lead to bleeding, fluid leakage, swelling, and scarring of the central retina, all of which may decrease vision. Wet AMD is always considered advanced AMD.

Symptoms: What You May Experience • In early dry AMD, there may be little to no change in vision. Over years, you may begin to notice gradual blurring of vision and increased difficulty going from brighter to darker environments, with your eyes taking longer to adjust. In advanced dry AMD, there may be a marked decrease in central vision, though this typically occurs gradually over time. In cases of wet AMD, however, vision

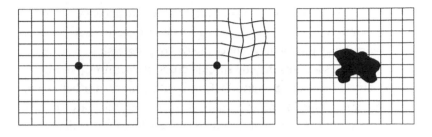

9.1. Left: normal Amsler grid. Center: distorted Amsler grid.
Right: blind spot in center of Amsler grid.

changes can be very sudden, with quick onset of blurry, distorted, or missing areas of central vision. AMD is painless.

Examination Findings: What the Doctor Looks For • Screening for AMD requires regular dilated eye exams, where your doctor examines the retina with lights and magnifying lenses. Often, a scan of the back of the eye, known as optical coherence tomography (OCT), takes a picture of the layers of the retina to evaluate the retinal deposits (drusen) and detect abnormal blood vessels. Other common tests include color photos, fundus autofluorescence, OCT angiography, and fluorescein angiography, where a dye that is injected into an arm vein to look for wet AMD. (One out of 225,000 people may be allergic to this dye.)

What You Can Do • There is no way to prevent AMD. Cigarette smoking, high cholesterol, high blood pressure, UV light, and cardiovascular disease are risk factors for AMD. To reduce your risk, management of these factors, in particular quitting smoking, is likely beneficial.

If you have early dry AMD, look at an Amsler grid, one eye at a time, each day or every few days to identify changes in vision, allowing for more prompt treatment if necessary. If you notice distortions or blind spots on the grid, call your eye doctor right away.

In addition to the Amsler grid, you can ask your eye doctor about a home tele-monitoring device that maps your field of vision to detect subtle changes. The device automatically sends results to a reading center for interpretation. If any concerning changes are found, the reading center would contact your eye doctor who would schedule an urgent visit to determine if you need treatment.

Treatment • For those with intermediate AMD, or advanced AMD in just one eye, a multivitamin formula called AREDS2 (Age Related Eye Disease Study 2) may moderately reduce the risk of progression to advanced AMD. AREDS2 vitamins include specific doses of vitamin C, vitamin E, copper, zinc, lutein, and zeaxanthin. Check with your doctor before taking another combination of "eye vitamins." Currently, there are no other proven treatments to prevent or reverse vision loss due to dry AMD, though significant research is ongoing.

For wet AMD, a class of medications known as "anti-VEGF" agents act against a protein that promotes abnormal blood vessel growth within the eye. They are administered by an injection into the vitreous of the eye, typically performed in the office. These injections are usually given repeatedly—as often as monthly—to help the abnormal blood vessels shrivel up and stop leaking and bleeding; this usually stabilizes the vision and may also lead to vision improvement. "Anti-VEGF" medications include ranibizumab (Lucentis), aflibercept (Eylea), bevacizumab (Avastin), and brolucizumab (Beovu). The specific medication used depends on a variety of factors and is best discussed with your doctor.

While the idea of receiving an injection into the eye may sound intimidating, it is a common and relatively safe procedure that is frequently performed in the office. The eye is numbed with eye drops or sometimes a numbing injection, and a cleaning drop is placed in the eye. An eyelid holder may be used to keep the eyelids open. A very fine short needle is inserted through the white of the eye (sclera) to inject a small amount of medication into the vitreous in the central part of the eye. The eyelid holder, if used, is removed. The whole procedure is typically quick and well tolerated with minimal discomfort. Risks include inflammation, bleeding, infection, and retinal tear/detachment; however, the risk is <1%. In some cases, laser treatment or surgery may be recommended if there has been a large amount of bleeding from the abnormal blood vessels.

In cases of irreversible central vision loss, there are numerous low vision aids and devices that have been developed to maximize your vision and enhance quality of life. These devices include magnifying lenses, telescopes, electronic magnifiers, and text-to-speech software. Low-vision therapy is often combined with these aids and teaches how to use these devices as well as adapt to changes in vision, so as to best preserve lifestyle and independence. Your eye doctor can refer you to a low-vision specialist to explore options and devices.

Prognosis: Will I See Better? • AMD is a common yet complex disease that has the potential to cause significant changes in central vision, affecting daily activities. Many with AMD do not experience vision loss, but for those who do, closely work with your eye doctor to develop a care plan that is best for you. Regular eye care, usually with a retina specialist, provides the best chance for preserving vision. While AMD can result in very blurry central vision, often in both eyes, it usually does not affect peripheral vision.

Additional Resources

https://www.aao.org/eye-health/diseases/amd-macular-degeneration
https://eyewiki.aao.org/Age-related_macular_degeneration

OBINNA UMUNAKWE, MD, PHD

What Is It? • Diabetic retinopathy is an eye disease that can develop from any type of diabetes, especially in those who have had diabetes for a long time or have poorly controlled diabetes. Almost 30% of those with diabetes over 40 years old have some degree of diabetic retinopathy. Diabetes can damage small blood vessels anywhere in the body. When this occurs in the retina of the eye, the result is diabetic retinopathy. Diabetic retinopathy has a nonproliferative stage and a more severe proliferative stage. In nonproliferative diabetic retinopathy, tiny damaged blood vessels break open, creating small spots of blood within the retina. Occasionally, fluid and other materials leak from damaged vessels causing retinal swelling. If swelling occurs in the macula of the retina, also known as diabetic macular edema, central vision may be affected.

Over time, proliferative diabetic retinopathy develops as areas of the retina become ischemic, or starved of blood supply and oxygen. The ischemic retinal tissue releases "feed-me" signals (vascular endothelial growth factor, or VEGF), and new abnormal retinal blood vessels, called neovascularization, grow and bleed. Bleeding into the vitreous, also known as vitreous hemorrhage, may cause sudden loss of vision. Scar tissue that grows with these new blood vessels can pull on and detach the retina, increasing the risk of permanent vision loss. Sometimes, neovascularization also occurs in the front portion of the eye and can cause glaucoma (neovascular glaucoma).

Symptoms: What You May Experience • Note that as your blood sugar fluctuates, your vision may fluctuate due to swelling of the lens within the eye; this is *not* diabetic retinopathy. Early stages of diabetic retinopathy are not typically associated with visual symptoms. This is why it is extremely important to have regular dilated eye exams to screen for diabetic retinopathy, if you have diabetes. Over time, you may experience blurred or distorted vision. In the proliferative stage, you may experience

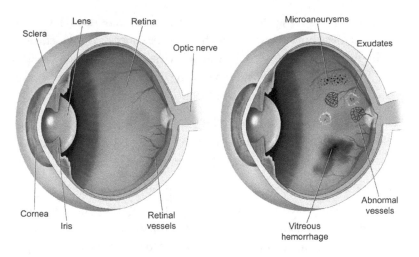

10.1. Left: normal retina. Right: retina affected by diabetic retinopathy.

dark floaters or loss of vision due to vitreous hemorrhage or retinal detachment, but sometimes there are no symptoms. If neovascular glaucoma develops, you may experience eye pain, blurry vision, headaches, and nausea from high eye pressures.

Examination Findings: What the Doctor Looks For • Examination findings vary depending on the stage of disease. Nonproliferative diabetic retinopathy examination findings may include few or many spots of blood in the retina, areas of retinal swelling including macular edema, retinal lipid deposits, and changes in the appearance of retinal veins and arteries. Proliferative diabetic retinopathy is characterized by neovascularization, which is the presence of fragile new abnormal blood vessels. Other possible examination findings in proliferative diabetic retinopathy include vitreous hemorrhage and tractional retinal detachment.

Your doctor may also obtain imaging studies such as photographs of the retina, optical coherence tomography (oct), or fluorescein angiography. oct allows your doctor to examine macular edema or ischemia in more detail. Fluorescein angiography helps to identify leaky blood vessels or areas of neovascularization.

What You Can Do • The most important step for reducing the risk of developing diabetic retinopathy is to maintain good control of your diabetes. This means working closely with your primary care doctor to keep your blood sugar under control. High blood pressure and high cholesterol should also be controlled. You should visit your eye doctor for diabetic retinopathy screening and monitoring at least yearly. More severe disease requires more frequent monitoring.

When to Call the Doctor • In addition to regularly scheduled visits, you should call the eye doctor if you experience decreased vision, loss of vision, new floaters, eye pain, or any vision symptoms.

Treatment • Prevention is key. Detecting diabetic retinopathy early is critical. Regular dilated eye examinations by an eye doctor are a must. Nonproliferative diabetic retinopathy generally does not require direct treatment aside from treating the underlying diabetes as well as high blood pressure and high cholesterol. If diabetic macular edema is present and causing visual changes, treatment options include injections of anti-VEGF or steroids into the eye, or laser treatment to the retina. Proliferative diabetic retinopathy is treated with laser therapy to reduce the amount of ischemic retinal tissue, which in turn, reduces the amount of VEGF production. Vitreous hemorrhage generally improves without intervention, but if it does not, vitrectomy surgery may be indicated. Retinal detachments due to traction are treated surgically. If neovascular glaucoma develops, it is treated with pressure-lowering eye drops, anti-VEGF injections, or glaucoma surgery depending on the severity.

Prognosis: Will I See Better? • Prognosis depends on the severity of the disease and the cause of reduced vision. Reduced vision due to diabetic retinopathy results from diabetic macular edema, retinal ischemia, vitreous hemorrhage, and/or retinal detachment. The vision can improve after resolution of diabetic macular edema or vitreous hemorrhage. Vision loss due to retinal ischemia may be permanent. Visual recovery after surgical repair of retinal detachment depends on the extent and chronicity of the detachment.

Additional Resources

https://www.aao.org/eye-health/diseases/what-is-diabetic-retinopathy
https://eyewiki.aao.org/Diabetic_Retinopathy

11 · Other Conditions of the Retina and Choroid

Hypertensive Retinopathy

DIANNA L. SELDOMRIDGE, MD, MBA

What Is It? • Hypertensive retinopathy is defined as the changes that occur in the retinal blood vessels and the retina as a result of hypertension (high blood pressure). Patients with hypertensive retinopathy are at risk for developing other eye diseases, the most common of which is a retinal vein occlusion. Less commonly, one may develop a retinal arterial macroaneurysm.

Symptoms: What You May Experience • There are varying degrees of hypertensive retinopathy, the mildest of which may not noticeably affect vision. Moderate to severe hypertensive retinopathy can lead to blurry vision or vision loss in one or both eyes due to bleeding, swelling, or ischemia (lack of blood flow and oxygen).

Examination Findings: What the Doctor Looks For • Your eye doctor will look for narrowing of the retinal arteries, compression of the retinal veins where arteries and veins cross, bleeding or swelling within the retina, swelling of the optic nerve, a weakening of the retinal arteries, and evidence of retinal artery blockage.

What You Can Do • The most important thing you can do is control your blood pressure with a low-salt diet, aerobic exercise, and medication if your primary care doctor prescribes it. You may need to ask your doctor if you are able to safely exercise.

When to Call the Doctor • Anytime you notice a change in your vision, you should make an appointment to see your eye doctor.

Treatment • If you develop hypertensive retinopathy, the best treatment is to control your blood pressure to prevent further damage. There are no eye drops, eye laser treatments, eye surgery, or glasses that can improve hypertensive retinopathy.

Prognosis: Will I See Better? • Vision loss that results from hypertensive retinopathy may be partially reversible. However, it may also become permanent, and therefore should be prevented by controlling your blood pressure.

Additional Resource

https://eyewiki.aao.org/Hypertensive_retinopathy

Retinal Artery Occlusion

MUGE R. KESEN, MD

What Is It? • The blood supply for the inner layers of the retina comes from a single artery, known as the central retinal artery, which is located at the back of the eye. A blockage of the central retinal artery or any of its branches in the retina leads to disruption of blood flow to the retina and is called a central or branch retinal artery occlusion.

Retinal artery occlusion can have a variety of causes. Most commonly, the artery is blocked by a small piece of debris flowing in the bloodstream. This debris often originates from the walls of diseased blood vessels elsewhere in the body. The debris can be a clot made up of platelets or an embolus made up of cholesterol or talc. Rarely, inflammation and swelling of the retinal artery itself can cause an artery occlusion.

When a retinal artery is blocked, the affected retina can no longer receive the oxygen and nourishment it needs to survive (called ischemia). If the blood supply is not restored within about 90 minutes, the retina in this area will begin to die. This may result in permanent loss of vision in that part of the eye.

Symptoms: What You May Experience • People who develop retinal artery occlusion will experience a sudden, often marked, decrease in their vision. The vision loss is usually painless and occurs over the course of seconds or minutes.

Examination Findings: What the Doctor Looks For • Your eye doctor will check your vision, which is often poor after a retinal artery occlusion. The doctor will also perform a dilated eye exam to examine the retina, which may appear white due to changes that occur following blockage of the artery. A fluorescein angiography (photographic dye test) may be performed to help identify where the occlusion has occurred.

What You Can Do • There is no definite way to prevent a retinal artery occlusion. However, since retinal artery occlusions are often a result of atherosclerotic (cholesterol) vessel disease in other parts of the body, working with your primary medical doctor to keep your blood pressure, blood sugar, cholesterol, and weight under control can help lower your risk of another occlusion in either eye.

When to Call the Doctor • Any time you experience sudden loss of vision, you should see your eye doctor as soon as possible.

Treatment • Although no treatment has proven effective in restoring vision after retinal artery occlusion, several therapies may sometimes be helpful. Your eye doctor may attempt to lower your eye pressure, which can occasionally help the blockage move farther downstream in the affected artery and allow for increased blood flow to certain parts of the retina. This may be done by massaging the eye gently, by using eye drops, or (sometimes) by removing a small amount of the fluid from the front part of the eye with a needle. If an embolus is identified during the eye examination, sometimes a retina specialist may laser it into smaller pieces to try to help improve blood flow in the affected retinal artery.

After a retinal artery occlusion, your eye doctor will monitor you periodically to make sure that you do not develop further complications such as the growth of abnormal blood vessels, which may result in increased eye pressure or bleeding within the eye. Patients with these complications may need to be treated with injections of medication into the eye or with a laser procedure.

Finding the underlying cause of a retinal artery occlusion is very important. Your primary medical doctor may perform other tests, such as an ultrasound of the arteries in your neck (carotid doppler) or echocardiogram of your heart, to look for a source of the embolus or the clot that may have blocked the artery. Older patients or those with autoimmune conditions may need blood tests to rule out inflammation of the blocked artery. Your primary medical doctor may also prescribe blood-thinning medications to lower your risk of future artery occlusions in the retina or in other parts of the body, including your brain and your heart.

Prognosis: Will I See Better? • The vision usually does not improve after a retinal artery occlusion, especially if a large part of the retina has lost its blood supply. In some cases, the vision may improve slightly.

Additional Resource

https://eyewiki.aao.org/Retinal_Artery_Occlusion

Branch Retinal Vein Occlusion (BRVO)

KIRIN KHAN, MD

What Is It? • The retina is a structure in the back of the eye responsible for converting light into signals that can be interpreted by the brain to produce images. Like any other part of the body, blood flows into the retina via an artery, called the central retinal artery. This central retinal artery brings nutrients, such as oxygen, to the retina. Once the retina has extracted what it needs from the blood, the blood flows back to the heart through the retinal veins. The central retinal vein is formed by the merging of smaller blood vessels known as the branch retinal veins.

Branch retinal vein occlusion (BRVO) occurs when there is a blockage in one of the branch retinal veins. This blockage may occur due to a blood clot in the vein or due to compression by an abnormally thickened adjacent retinal artery. Blocked retinal veins restrict the normal pattern of blood flow, which can have two consequences. First, the retina experiences decreased access to blood and the vital nutrients it carries, such as oxygen. Second, the occluded branch retinal veins may begin to leak fluid and blood, resulting in swelling and bleeding within the retina. Occasionally, decreased blood flow within the retina may lead to the growth of new abnormal blood vessels, called neovascularization. These blood vessels have an abnormal structure and may leak fluid or bleed, causing further retinal damage and vision loss.

Symptoms: What You May Experience • The macula is the center portion of the retina where light is focused to ultimately provide sharp, detailed vision. If the occluded branch retinal vein cannot drain blood from the macula, the macula may develop fluid buildup and swelling, known as macular edema, as well as ischemia or lack of blood flow around the area. This may result in painless blurring, graying, or loss of vision in the affected area. Vision changes can occur suddenly over a period of minutes or more gradually over a period of hours to days. If the occluded branch retinal vein does not supply the macula, it is possible that no symptoms will be noted since the macula has not been affected. BRVO usually only occurs in one eye but may develop in both eyes.

Examination Findings: What the Doctor Looks For • Your eye doctor may perform a dilated eye exam to check for swelling of the retina (edema), bleeding within the retina, or growth of new abnormal blood vessels (neovascularization). Additionally, the doctor may perform imaging tests such as fluorescein angiography, optical coherence tomography (OCT), or OCT angiography (OCT-A). In fluorescein angiography, a dye is injected into a vein in the arm, which then travels to the eye; a special camera captures images of the retina as the dye flows through it. This test may show if any veins are occluded, if retinal edema is present, or if retinal neovascularization has occurred. OCT is a non-invasive scan that can be used to better assess if there is swelling in the retina by showing a detailed view of the different layers of the retina. OCT-A can map out the retinal blood vessels without using an intravenous dye.

If you are under the age of 50 and do not have high blood pressure, your doctor may send you for blood tests to look for other causes of the BRVO.

What You Can Do • Typically BRVO affects patients over 50 with high blood pressure, diabetes, glaucoma, or hardening of the arteries (arteriosclerosis). To lower the risk of developing BRVO, monitor your blood pressure with your primary medical doctor, follow a healthy diet, exercise regularly, and do not smoke, as smoking increases the risk of arterial hardening. Additionally, regular eye pressure checks are important because increased eye pressure, which may be related to glaucoma, can contribute to the development of BRVO. Regular dilated eye exams and visual acuity checks can also help detect asymptomatic BRVO.

Patients with BRVO should continue to monitor the factors named above since there is a 10% risk of developing any retinal vein occlusion in the other eye over a 3-year period.

When to Call the Doctor • Any vision loss or vision changes warrants urgent medical attention. Patients with known BRVO should seek care if their vision worsens or if they begin to experience any visual symptoms in either eye.

Treatment • Treatment of BRVO focuses on reducing the side effects of the blocked retinal vein as opposed to actually eliminating the blockage. Eyes with BRVO but no macular edema may be observed closely without treatment. Patients with BRVO and associated macular edema may undergo laser treatment or injections of medications known as anti-vascular endothelial growth factor (anti-VEGF) drugs, such as bevacizumab (Avastin), ranibizumab (Lucentis), and aflibercept (Eylea). These medications are injected into the vitreous cavity in the back of the eye, usually monthly, to decrease swelling and bleeding in the retina as these complications may worsen vision. These injections are very safe and have a less than 1% risk of infection and bleeding and more rarely, retinal detachment. Eyes that do not respond to anti-VEGF medications may be given steroid injections such as preservative-free triamcinolone (Triesence); however, steroid injected in or around the eye can contribute to cataract growth and also elevated eye pressure. Therefore, steroids are often used carefully in eyes with glaucoma.

Some eyes with BRVO may develop retinal neovascularization. These abnormal blood vessels can leak contents (hemorrhage) and cause further retinal damage and vision loss. Laser and sometimes anti-VEGF injections may be used to treat and prevent further neovascularization.

Prognosis: Will I See Better? • Without treatment, 1/3 get better, 1/3 remain the same, and 1/3 worsen. It is not possible to predict which eyes may improve; however, most will experience some vision improvement over time. Others may not experience visual improvement. Eyes that are treated earlier often have better visual outcomes.

Additional Resources

https://eyewiki.aao.org/Branch_retinal_vein_occlusion

https://www.aao.org/eye-health/diseases/branch-retinal-vein-occlusion
    -treatment

https://www.asrs.org/patients/retinal-diseases/24/branch-retinal-vein-occlusion

Central Retinal Vein Occlusion (CRVO)

KIRIN KHAN, MD

What Is It? • The retina is a structure in the back of the eye responsible for converting light into signals that can be interpreted by the brain to produce images. The retina has one main artery named the central retinal artery that brings blood and nutrients to it. Similarly, the central retinal vein carries blood away from the retina back to the heart. In central retinal vein occlusion (CRVO), a blockage occurs in the central retinal vein, restricting the venous outflow of blood. This may lead to inadequate nutrients reaching the retina, as well as leakage of fluid and blood, resulting in swelling and bleeding within the retina. Occasionally, decreased blood flow to the retina may lead to neovascularization, or the growth of new abnormal blood vessels. These blood vessels have an abnormal structure and may leak fluid or blood, causing further retinal damage and vision loss.

There are several theories regarding the underlying process that leads to blood clot formation within the central retinal vein. The first theory suggests that when the central retinal vein is compressed, there is a change in blood flow that promotes the formation of an occlusive blood clot. Another theory suggests that the central retinal vein may experience direct compression by the adjacent central retinal artery when it becomes stiff due to cholesterol plaque buildup in the artery wall. Lastly, the normal blood flow in the central retinal vein may be impeded in patients with high eye pressure, which may be related to glaucoma.

Symptoms: What You May Experience • Vision changes in one eye can occur suddenly over a period of minutes or more gradually over a period of hours to days. Unlike BRVO, which may be asymptomatic, patients with CRVO usually report some degree of vision change. CRVO typically occurs in one eye but in 1% of people it may affect both eyes. Blockage of the central retinal vein causes fluid and blood to leak out of the vein, leading to swelling and bleeding within the retina. If the macula (central part of the retina) is affected, you may experience painless blurring, graying, or loss of vision.

Examination Findings: What the Doctor Looks For • An eye doctor will perform a dilated eye exam to check for swelling of the retina (edema), bleeding within the retina, or neovascularization. Additionally, the doctor may perform imaging tests such as fluorescein angiography, optical coherence tomography (OCT), or OCT angiography (OCT-A). In fluorescein angiography, a dye is injected into a vein in the arm, which then travels to the eye; a special camera captures images of the retina as the dye flows through it. (One in 225,000 people are allergic to fluorescein.) This test may show if the central retinal vein is occluded, if retinal edema is present, or if retinal neovascularization has occurred. OCT is a noninvasive scan that can be used to better assess if there is swelling in the retina by showing a detailed view of the different layers of the retina. OCT-A is a non-invasive way to map out the blood vessels without getting intravenous fluorescein.

Patients with CRVO who are under the age of 50, especially without high blood pressure or glaucoma, may be tested for blood clotting factors and genetic defects in their blood clotting system.

What You Can Do • Several conditions can contribute to the formation of CRVO. These include but are not limited to high blood pressure, high cholesterol, diabetes, and increased eye pressure (glaucoma). Regular appointments with a primary care physician and your eye doctor for early detection of these conditions is recommended. Additionally, a healthy diet and regular exercise can help prevent the conditions that contribute to CRVO.

Patients with CRVO should continue to monitor their blood pressure, cholesterol, diabetes, and/or glaucoma as these conditions contribute to the 1% risk per year for development of CRVO in the other eye.

When to Call the Doctor • Any changes in or loss of vision warrants urgent medical attention by an eye doctor. Patients with known CRVO should seek care if their vision worsens or their eye becomes painful.

Treatment • Treatment of CRVO focuses on reducing the side effects of the blocked retinal vein as opposed to actually eliminating the blockage. Eyes with CRVO but no macular edema may be observed closely without treatment. Eyes with CRVO and associated macular edema may receive injections into the vitreous of the eye of medications known as anti-VEGF drugs, such as bevacizumab (Avastin), ranibizumab (Lucentis), or aflibercept (Eylea). These medications are injected into the vitreous of the eye, usually monthly, to decrease swelling and bleeding in the retina as these complications may worsen vision. Eyes that do not respond to anti-VEGF drugs may be given steroid injections in or around the eye.

Occasionally, eyes with CRVO can develop neovascularization. Earlier detection of these abnormal blood vessels is important; these blood vessels can leak contents (hemorrhage and fluid) and cause further retinal damage and vision loss. Abnormal new blood vessels on the iris and in the angle of the eye can result in high eye pressure, called neovascular glaucoma. Laser treatment and anti-VEGF injections may be needed to treat and prevent further neovascularization.

Prognosis: Will I See Better? • The vision rarely improves in untreated eyes with CRVO and sometimes it may worsen. With treatment, the vision will likely improve in most eyes but it is not possible to predict how much improvement the eye may experience. Earlier treatment is recommended.

Additional Resources

https://www.aao.org/eye-health/diseases/central-retinal-vein-occlusion-diagnosis

https://www.asrs.org/patients/retinal-diseases/22/central-retinal-vein-occlusion

https://eyewiki.aao.org/Central_Retinal_Vein_Occlusion

Cystoid Macular Edema

CASON ROBBINS, BS

What Is It? • Cystoid macular edema (CME) is a condition in which fluid from retinal blood vessels leaks into the macula, the central part of the retina. The fluid accumulates in small pockets, known as cystoid spaces, inside the retina. This fluid causes the retina to swell, which can affect vision in that eye. CME is not a disease itself, but may be associated with many different eye diseases. One common cause of CME develops after uncomplicated cataract surgery, but it may also occur in eyes with other conditions such as diabetic retinopathy, retinal vein occlusion, inflammation in the eye, and other eye surgeries.

Symptoms: What You May Experience • You may notice painless blurring, graying, or distortion of vision (for instance, straight lines may appear wavy). When CME happens after cataract surgery, patients may initially have improved vision right after surgery followed by slowly worsening vision over several weeks afterward. Some patients who have CME do not notice a significant decrease in their vision.

Examination Findings: What the Doctor Looks For • Your eye doctor will perform a dilated eye exam to examine the retina for any swelling within the macula. Other imaging tests, including fluorescein angiography or optical coherence tomography (OCT), may be used to confirm the presence of CME. Your doctor may also look for signs and perform tests to check for other eye conditions that could be causing CME.

What You Can Do • The best way to try to prevent the development of CME is to make sure that other diseases that may affect the eye, such as diabetes and high blood pressure, are under control and that you are following your doctor's advice for treating these conditions. In some situations, your cataract surgeon may suggest using nonsteroidal anti-inflammatory drugs (NSAIDs) before and after cataract surgery to decrease the risk of CME.

When to Call the Doctor • If you experience blurry or distorted vision, you should contact your eye doctor. Although CME may be the cause of these changes, your doctor will also check for other potentially serious causes of visual loss or distortion.

Treatment • CME can be treated in a variety of ways depending on its cause. After eye surgery, eye drops such as steroids or NSAID medications are often used. These eye drops have to be used for at least 3 months to assess their effectiveness. Steroid eye drops sometimes may cause the eye pressure to become elevated while using the drop. In other cases, one or more injections of medication, such as steroid or anti-vascular endothelial growth factor (anti-VEGF), into the vitreous cavity of or around the eye may be suggested. Rarely, laser therapy or eye surgery may be needed as part of the treatment for CME.

Prognosis: Will I See Better? • Visual prognosis for CME depends on the cause and severity. CME after cataract surgery has an excellent chance of improving on its own or with medications. CME from other causes has a variable visual outcome, although some improvement in eyesight can be expected with decreased swelling in the macula. Improvement is often gradual and can take several months. Long-standing CME can sometimes lead to permanently decreased vision, which may not improve even after the CME goes away.

Central Serous Chorioretinopathy

ABHILASH GUDURU, MD

What Is It? • Central serous chorioretinopathy (CSCR) is a condition in which fluid leaks and accumulates under the macula, the central part of the retina. It typically occurs between the ages of 20 and 50 and is up to 10 times more common in males. The cause of CSCR is unknown, but there have been some associations with stress, "type A personality," high blood pressure, pregnancy, and the use of any type of steroid, including testosterone. In most cases, the fluid spontaneously reabsorbs over weeks to months, and the vision improves. Usually only one eye is affected; however, CSCR can recur in the same eye or affect the other eye. Rarely, CSCR may be associated with choroidal neovascularization, a more serious condition in which abnormal blood vessels grow underneath the retina.

Symptoms: What You May Experience • You may notice the sudden or gradual onset of painless, blurry vision or a blind spot in the center of your vision. Other symptoms may include decreased color saturation or visual distortion such that objects may appear smaller than usual or straight lines may appear wavy.

Examination Findings: What the Doctor Looks For • A dilated eye exam will often reveal an area of retinal thickening related to leakage of fluid. A photographic dye test called fluorescein angiography or a retinal scan called optical coherence tomography (OCT) may also be performed to confirm the diagnosis of CSCR and rule out other conditions.

What You Can Do • There is little you can do to hasten the resolution of CSCR. To prevent CSCR, avoiding steroids of any kind is important. If you are using inhaled, topical, or systemic steroid medications, check with your medical doctor to see if another medication could be substituted instead. Attempting to reduce your stress level may help, but there is no proven benefit to addressing this.

When to Call the Doctor • If you experience decreased vision or distortion, you should contact your eye doctor. Although CSCR may be the cause, there are many other potentially serious causes of visual loss or distortion.

Treatment • CSCR usually resolves on its own and does not require specific treatment. If CSCR is not resolving, is recurrent, or involves both eyes, treatment is often indicated. Oral acetazolamide (500 mg twice a day) can sometimes hasten reabsorption of the fluid. Some studies suggest that certain blood pressure–lowering medications such as oral eplerenone and spironolactone may aid in recovery; it is important that your eye doctor or primary doctor monitor your blood potassium levels if these medications are used. If a specific leak is identified on fluorescein angiography, eyes with chronic CSCR may benefit from focal laser treatment to that leak; however, laser has potential risks and does not necessarily lead to a better final visual outcome. Another type of laser called photodynamic therapy (PDT) with intravenous verteporfin, a specialized laser-activated medication, may be another treatment option in some cases. If PDT is used, you must stay out of direct sunlight for up to 5 days.

Prognosis: Will I See Better? • In 80–90% of cases, nearly full visual recovery occurs over several months, although some mild residual symptoms may be expected. A small number of patients will have multiple recurrences, which may lead to a permanent decrease in central vision over time.

Posterior Vitreous Detachment/Flashes and Floaters

PARAMJIT K. BHULLAR, MD

What Is It? • The human eye has two main compartments: the anterior segment (front of the eye) and the posterior segment (back of the eye). The vitreous gel is a clear substance that fills a large volume of the posterior segment. At birth, the vitreous is attached to the retina, a neurosensory tissue that lines the back of the eye. With increasing age, the vitreous naturally liquefies, collapses, and separates from the retina in a process called posterior vitreous detachment (PVD). This is a normal process of aging but can occur earlier in nearsighted eyes, after eye surgery or injury, or due to other eye conditions. A PVD occurs gradually, often evolving over several weeks to months, and may occur in one eye first or both eyes simultaneously.

Symptoms: What You May Experience • The vitreous often detaches from the retina without issue, in which case you may be completely asymptomatic or may notice one or several floaters. These floaters are often the result of shadows cast by areas of condensed vitreous and may be described as strings, lines, dots, or fuzzy particles that float around in your visual field. However, vitreous detachment can also lead to tugging on the retina, particularly in areas of firm attachment, and you may notice flashing lights in the eye, even when the eye is closed. If the tugging on the retina is forceful enough, it can cause a retinal break. Fluid can creep into this retinal break and under the retina and cause the retina to detach from the eye wall. In the event of a retinal break with a detachment, you may experience an increase in the number of floaters, the presence of flashing lights, or a sensation of a curtain or veil coming over your vision in that eye from any direction.

Examination Findings: What the Doctor Looks For • The eye doctor will do a complete eye exam, including a vision check and dilated eye exam. Your doctor will evaluate the vitreous gel to see if a separation from the retina has occurred and will also check for any evidence of a retinal break or detachment. Occasionally, the eye doctor may need to press on the eyelid or eye with a cotton tip or other instrument to see the entire retina. Your doctor may also order some imaging tests such as an optical coherence tomography (OCT) scan, which may show where the vitreous and retinal surfaces are in relation to one another.

What You Can Do • There is nothing one can do to prevent or slow down a PVD; it is considered a normal part of the aging process. Certain individuals at a higher risk for retinal detachment, such as those with a high degree of nearsightedness (prescriptions of −6 diopters or more) or a family history of retinal detachment should be aware of the symptoms associated with a retinal break or detachment. It is very important to seek urgent eye care if you develop these symptoms, as prompt treatment or surgery for a retinal break or detachment may prevent significant vision loss.

When to Call the Doctor • If you notice increased flashing lights, floaters, a curtain or veil coming over your vision, or any other visual changes, it is important to seek a prompt eye evaluation.

Treatment • In cases of a retinal break(s) without retinal detachment, a laser procedure or freezing treatment (cryotherapy) may be necessary to tack down the retina to prevent a retinal detachment. If you develop a retinal detachment, time-sensitive surgery may be necessary to help reattach the retina. If no retinal breaks or detachments are present, no intervention is needed. However, patients with an evolving PVD remain at high risk for developing a retinal break or detachment and should be monitored closely after the initial onset of symptoms.

Prognosis: Will I See Better? • Over time, floaters related to uncomplicated PVD usually float out of the vision, become smaller, and are less noticeable; central visual acuity is generally not affected. For those with a retinal break(s) or detachment, prompt treatment may help prevent severe vision loss.

Additional Resources

https://www.aao.org/eye-health/diseases/what-are-symptoms-of-pvd

https://eyewiki.aao.org/Posterior_vitreous_detachment

Vitreomacular Adhesion and Vitreomacular Traction

CHRISTOPHER SUN, MBBS AND

DANIEL S. W. TING, MD, PHD

What Is It? • Vitreomacular adhesion (VMA) and vitreomacular traction (VMT) are conditions that arise due to abnormal attachments between the vitreous gel and the retina, which line the back of the eye. At birth, the vitreous gel in the eye is firmly attached to the retina. This vitreous liquefies and condenses with age, often separating from the retina in a process called posterior vitreous detachment. However, sometimes the gel remains attached to the macula (the center part of the retina) and can distort the normal anatomy of the retina. In VMA, the vitreous gel and retina remain adherent, but there is no traction, or tugging, on the retina. In contrast, VMT is characterized by incomplete separation of the vitreous gel from the retina with the presence of retinal traction and distortion; this abnormal traction can sometimes progress to form a hole in the retina, called a macular hole.

Symptoms: What You May Experience • If the degree of retinal distortion is mild, you may be completely asymptomatic. If there is more significant retinal distortion or a macular hole, you may experience painless blurring of vision, blind spots, or metamorphopsia (straight lines appear wavy). Symptoms are gradual and usually only one eye is affected.

Examination Findings: What the Doctor Looks For • Your eye doctor will dilate your eye and perform a careful retinal examination, which may reveal a cellophane-like membrane over the macula called an epiretinal membrane. Optical coherence tomography (OCT), a non-invasive imaging test, may be performed to better visualize the abnormal vitreous attachment and the extent of distortion.

What You Can Do • There is nothing you can do to prevent the development of VMA or VMT. For VMA or mild VMT, there is usually nothing that needs to be done by your eye doctor. For more severe VMT or a macular hole, your eye doctor will often discuss the available treatment options.

When to Call the Doctor • If you experience decreased vision, blind spots, or distortion of vision you should contact your eye doctor immediately.

Treatment • For VMA or mild VMT, observation is usually recommended as approximately one-third of eyes will experience spontaneous resolution of the condition. For severe VMT, there are several methods of treatment, which may include injecting a gas bubble into the vitreous cavity of the eye or retinal surgery to remove the vitreous gel (vitrectomy). Success rates are generally high, especially with vitrectomy surgery; however, there is a 1% risk of complications with these treatments. Rarely, consideration of a single injection of ocriplasmin (Jetrea) can be explored to release the VMA or VMT in symptomatic eyes; however, the success rate is low, and there is a risk of short-term, often temporary, vision loss. Your retinal specialist will go through each procedure to determine what method of treatment is the most suitable for you.

Prognosis: Will I See Better? • In the majority of cases, there will be some improvement in vision and symptoms (e.g., central distortion) with treatment, provided the underlying retina is healthy. There is, however, a very small chance that your vision may remain the same or get worse despite treatment. In addition, should any complication from the treatment occur, this may affect your final visual outcome.

Additional Resource

https://eyewiki.aao.org/Vitreomacular_Traction_Syndrome

Macular Hole

MUGE R. KESEN, MD

What Is It? • The macula is the center part of the retina and is responsible for detailed central vision. A macular hole is a small, full-thickness break in the center of the retina within the macula. Macular holes are usually age-related and develop in otherwise healthy patients over the age of 60. However, they can also occur due to trauma or other eye diseases. Typically, a macular hole occurs in only one eye, but about 10–15% of patients may develop a macular hole in the other eye over their lifetime.

Symptoms: What You May Experience • In the early stages of a macular hole, people may notice a slight distortion or blurriness in their central vision. In later stages with a full-thickness macular hole, there will likely be a central round blind spot.

Examination Findings: What the Doctor Looks For • The eye doctor may ask you to look at an Amsler grid with a central dot in the middle and describe what you can and cannot see on that grid. Some of the lines may be missing or distorted, and you may not be able to see the central dot if you have a full-thickness macular hole. The eye doctor will perform a dilated eye exam to directly visualize the macular hole. They may also perform a non-invasive imaging test called optical coherence tomography (OCT) to visualize the macular hole in cross-section.

What You Can Do • There is no proven way to prevent the development of a macular hole. You should be aware of its symptoms so that if a macular hole develops, you can be examined by an eye doctor in a timely manner and undergo treatment if necessary.

When to Call the Doctor • If you begin to notice distortion in the central vision of one of your eyes, or if straight lines begin to look wavy, you should contact your eye doctor for an examination. Some patients who have developed a macular hole in one eye will periodically test their other eye at home with an Amsler grid given to them by their eye doctor.

Treatment • Although some macular holes can (rarely) close spontaneously, almost all of them will need to be treated. There are no eye drops, pills, injections, or laser procedures to treat a macular hole. An injection of ocriplasmin (Jetrea) may sometimes be used in eyes with smaller macular holes that have the vitreous gel still attached to the hole but the success rates are not high and there are significant although uncommon visual risks. The most common treatment for a full-thickness macular hole is vitrectomy, a type of retinal surgery in which the vitreous gel inside the eye is removed to release traction and close the hole. The surgeon may also inject a gas bubble into the eye during the surgery and ask you to remain face down for up to one week after surgery to position the gas bubble against the macular hole to help it heal. The gas bubble will dissolve by itself over time and be replaced by your own eye fluid.

While the gas bubble is in the eye, the vision is often poor. Also, it is critical not to fly in an airplane, travel to areas at high altitudes, or lie flat in a supine position (i.e., on your back). Also, if you were to undergo another surgery while a gas bubble is in your eye, it is critical that the anesthesiologist and doctor or dentist know about the gas bubble in your eye so that the anesthetics can be adjusted appropriately. You may be provided with a wristband indicating the presence of gas in your eye and be asked to wear it until your eye doctor has confirmed that the gas bubble has reabsorbed and is no longer present. Sometimes your surgeon may opt to use a silicone oil bubble that would allow you to change altitudes and receive any type of anesthetic but it requires another eye surgery to remove the silicone oil and may have lower macular hole closure rates so silicone oil is less commonly used.

Prognosis: Will I See Better? • Without surgery, you will likely not experience any improvement in your vision. Vitrectomy surgery successfully closes a macular hole in over 90% of cases. When the hole is closed, most will experience stabilization or improvement in central vision. If

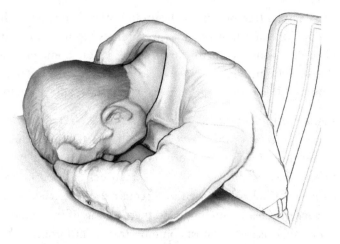

11.1. Some retinal surgeries require the patient to be positioned face down for several days afterward.

you have had a macular hole for less than six months, you may have a better chance of recovering vision than if the macular hole has been present for a longer period.

If you have not previously had cataract surgery, then you are likely to develop a worsening cataract within months to years after macular hole surgery and will ultimately need cataract surgery for full restoration of vision.

Additional Resources

https://www.aao.org/eye-health/diseases/what-is-macular-hole
https://eyewiki.aao.org/Macular_Hole

Epiretinal Membrane

JAMES H. POWERS, MD

What Is It? • An epiretinal membrane is a thin sheet of fibrous tissue that develops over the central portion of the retina called the macula. Also known as macular pucker, cellophane retinopathy, or preretinal gliosis, this thin film may sometimes cause distortion of vision. An epiretinal membrane forms when glial cells on the retinal surface grow into a membranous sheet. The development of an epiretinal membrane is most commonly associated with a posterior vitreous detachment or a retinal break, but often no specific cause is identified. Sometimes they may occur after retinal detachment, eye trauma, inflammation/infection, or retinal blood vessel abnormalities.

Symptoms: What You May Experience • Mild epiretinal membranes are often asymptomatic. However, if the epiretinal membrane is relatively thick or distorts the anatomy of the macula of the retina, you may experience painless visual blurring or distortion. Often, straight lines may appear wavy. Vision changes may be progressive over time in 10% of people. It is not possible to become completely blind from an epiretinal membrane itself.

Examination Findings: What the Doctor Looks For • Your eye doctor will check your vision and dilate your eyes to examine the retina for an epiretinal membrane. Often a non invasive retinal imaging technique called optical coherence tomography (OCT) will be used to assist in the diagnosis. Fluorescein angiography, a photographic dye test, may also be performed. (One in 225,000 people are allergic to intravenous fluorescein.)

What You Can Do • There are no known ways to prevent the formation of an epiretinal membrane.

When to Call the Doctor • An epiretinal membrane is often diagnosed incidentally. If you are experiencing decreased or distorted vision, you should contact your eye doctor for a comprehensive eye exam.

Treatment • As longs as it is not worsening or significantly affecting your vision, most epiretinal membranes may simply be monitored by your eye doctor. In some cases, specialized retinal surgery may be required. This retinal surgery involves removal of the vitreous gel (vitrectomy) and peeling of the epiretinal membrane. This surgery can lead to the development of a cataract in the affected eye and there is about a 1% risk of other complications such as bleeding, infection, and retinal detachment.

Prognosis: Will I See Better? • If surgical intervention is not required, your epiretinal membrane is likely mild and not significantly affecting your vision. For those with more severe epiretinal membranes, vitrectomy surgery may result in some visual recovery in the following months and may continue to improve up to 1 year after surgery. The vision will likely not recover back to "normal."

Additional Resources

https://www.asrs.org/patients/retinal-diseases/19/epiretinal-membranes
https://eyewiki.aao.org/Epiretinal_Membrane

Retinal Detachment

KIM JIRAMONGKOLCHAI, MD

What Is It? • The retina is a light-sensing tissue that lines the back of the eyeball and transmits visual information to the optic nerve which travels to the brain. A retinal detachment is the separation of the retina from its normal position lining the back of the eye. When this happens, the retina cannot properly function. Depending on the area of the retina that is detached, partial or central visual loss can occur. Without prompt treatment, permanent vision loss may result.

The most common cause of retinal detachment is a break, which can be a tear or a hole, in the retina that allows fluid inside the vitreous cavity of the eye to enter and track underneath the retina, detaching it. Other less common types of retinal detachment are tractional, which results from scar tissue on the surface of the retina contracting and mechanically pulling the retina away from the wall of the eye, and exudative, which is a result of inflammation leading to fluid accumulation under the retina without the presence of a retinal break.

Retinal detachment is more likely to occur in those with nearsightedness (myopia), a history of previous retinal breaks or detachments in either eye, prior eye surgeries, prior eye trauma, or a family history of retinal detachment.

Symptoms: What You May Experience • Symptoms of a retinal break can include a sudden or gradual increase in flashes of light or floaters, which look like "fireworks" and "cobwebs" or spots that float in the field of vision. When the retina detaches, additional symptoms include a dark curtain or shade that may be seen coming over the vision from any side. There is no pain associated with a retinal break or detachment.

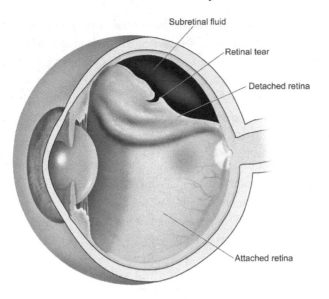

11.2. Retinal detachment.

Examination Findings: What the Doctor Looks For • Your eye doctor will check your central and peripheral vision and perform a complete dilated eye exam to look for any retinal breaks or detachments.

What You Can Do • There is nothing you can do to prevent a retinal break or detachment other than avoiding eye injury and knowing the associated risk factors and symptoms so that you may seek prompt eye care.

When to Call the Doctor • It is important to call your eye doctor immediately if you notice new flashing lights, floaters, decreased vision, or a dark curtain or shade covering any part of your vision from any direction. Early treatment of a retinal break may prevent a retinal detachment. Prompt treatment of a retinal detachment may prevent significant vision loss.

Treatment • Retinal breaks without a detachment may be treated by a retina specialist in the outpatient office with laser therapy or cryotherapy (freezing). Retinal detachments are usually treated with either an office-based procedure or retinal surgery in the operating room depending on the type, location, and severity of the retinal detachment. If the central vision (macula) is not involved in the retinal detachment, it is often re-paired within 24 hours or so. If the central vision is involved in the retinal detachment, the retina is often repaired within 7 days of when the central vision became involved. If the central vision has been involved in the retinal detachment more than 7 days, the retina can be repaired on the next available surgery day. The following are various methods that may be used to repair certain types of retinal detachments:

PNEUMATIC RETINOPEXY Cryotherapy is performed to the edges of the retinal break after which a gas bubble is injected into the vitreous cavity of the eye. You may then be asked to position your head in a certain direction to maximize coverage of the gas bubble over the retinal break. This procedure is suitable for select patients with certain types of detachments and is done in the office.

SCLERAL BUCKLE SURGERY A hard silicone band is placed around the white of the eye to indent the eye wall and support the retinal break externally. You will not be able to see the scleral buckle in the mirror or in your vision. With this surgery, it is expected that the eye will become slightly more nearsighted; however, this can often be corrected with a change in glasses or contact lens prescription. There is a small risk of double vision with this procedure, which usually resolves within a few weeks. The hard silicone band stays there forever and is not magnetic. This surgery is performed in the operating room. Sometimes a gas bubble is also used to hold the retina in place while it heals. It is important not to fly in an airplane or receive certain types of anesthetics while the gas bubble is in place.

VITRECTOMY SURGERY The vitreous gel is removed, and the retina is reattached after the fluid underneath the retina is drained and the retinal breaks are treated. A gas bubble or silicone oil bubble is used in this surgery to help hold the retina in place. If gas is used, you may be asked to position your head in a certain direction to maximize the coverage of the gas bubble over the retinal tear. It is also important for the patient to avoid flying or traveling to high altitudes as the gas bubble will expand within the eye. If additional surgery needs to be performed while the gas bubble is in the eye, the patient should notify their anesthesiologist as certain anesthetics can interfere with the gas bubble. The gas bubble will slowly dissolve by itself and be replaced by your own eye fluid. Silicone oil may be used on select types of retinal detachments and in those who cannot position properly. If silicone oil is used, a separate surgery will be required to remove it. Reattachment of the retina is successful in 85–90% of cases after a single surgery; however, 10–15% may require additional surgeries due to the formation of scar tissue (proliferative vitreoretinopathy) that causes the retina to re-detach. After vitrectomy, cataracts tend to worsen in the following months to years, and cataract surgery will likely be required at a later date.

Prognosis: Will I See Better?

Most recover significant vision after the retina is reattached. However, you may not recover to your baseline vision, especially if the central portion of the retina called the macula was detached.

Additional Resources

https://nei.nih.gov/learn-about-eye-health/eye-conditions-and-diseases/
retinal-detachment
https://www.aao.org/eye-health/diseases/detached-torn-retina
https://eyewiki.aao.org/Retinal_Detachment

Proliferative Vitreoretinopathy

ANANTH SASTRY, MD

What Is It? • Proliferative vitreoretinopathy (PVR) is the formation of scar tissue on or under the retina. This occurs as a result of a full thickness retinal break in an eye with a retinal detachment. The break in the retina allows cells and pigment that are normally behind the retina to move forward into the vitreous gel. This results in a complex inflammatory reaction that allows scar tissue to form.

PVR occurs in about 10% of eyes with a retinal detachment, and it is more likely to occur if the retinal detachment happened weeks to months before being repaired. Other risk factors for PVR development include younger age, hemorrhage, eye trauma, prior eye surgery, or prior eye infections.

Symptoms: What You May Experience • Sometimes there are no symptoms of PVR. In other cases, the scar tissue that characterizes PVR can contract and pull against the retina, leading to blurred or distorted vision. PVR may also cause the retina to re-detach after surgical repair and may be associated with flashing lights, floaters, or the sensation of a "curtain" coming over your field of vision from any side.

Examination Findings: What the Doctor Looks For • Your eye doctor will perform a full eye exam, including a dilated eye exam, to look for areas with abnormal scar tissue, retinal breaks, or retinal detachment. Your doctor will also check your vision and eye pressure, since PVR may also damage the ciliary body, a structure responsible for secreting fluid that keeps the eye pressurized.

What You Can Do • Although there are risk factors for the formation of PVR as outlined above, there is nothing you can do to actively prevent it.

When to Call the Doctor • You should call the eye doctor if you develop new flashing lights, new floaters, changes in vision, or eye pain.

Treatment • The only way that existing PVR membranes can be removed is through vitrectomy surgery by a retina specialist. The surgeon will remove the vitreous gel from the eye, peel any scar tissue causing traction on the retina, and in severe cases, may even make relaxing cuts in the retina to minimize traction and the chance of a recurrent retinal detachment. The surgeon may also place a hard silicone scleral buckle around the white part of the eye (sclera) to provide better stability to the retina.

In addition to the above procedures, the surgeon may also need to remove the crystalline lens and place a silicone oil bubble into the eye to help the retina reattach. This oil may need to stay in the eye for months to years depending on the severity of the detachment. The oil can then be removed from the eye at a later time as part of a followup surgery. After the surgery, the surgeon may have you position your head in a particular manner to help the retina reattach.

After surgery to remove PVR membranes and reattach the retina, some retina surgeons may also consider methotrexate injections into the silicone-oil-filled vitreous cavity of the eye to decrease the risk of recurrent PVR. This involves injecting about 0.1 milliliters, or 400 micrograms, of methotrexate into the vitreous cavity each week for about 8–12 weeks and then every other week for 4 weeks. It is important to keep the eye surface well lubricated if methotrexate injections are used.

Prognosis: Will I See Better? • You may gain some vision back after the PVR scar tissue has been removed and the retina has been reattached. However, this visual improvement may be limited and is unlikely to be at the level that you had prior to developing PVR.

Additional Resource

https://en.wikipedia.org/wiki/Proliferative_vitreoretinopathy

Retinitis Pigmentosa and Other Hereditary Retinal Degenerations

ALESSANDRO IANNACCONE, MD, MS, FARVO

What Is It? • There are many inherited eye diseases that can lead to progressive retinal damage. All of these disorders are inherited, meaning that they are passed to a child through genetic changes carried by one or both parents. Due to different inheritance patterns, the parents of an affected individual may or may not be symptomatic and these diseases can skip generations. Retinitis pigmentosa (RP) and cone-rod dystrophy (CORD) are two main groups of retinal degenerations. Those that predominantly affect the macula are termed macular dystrophies. Some retinal dystrophies can be associated with other systemic problems such as hearing loss, obesity, and kidney problems. When these findings or conditions occur simultaneously, they are called "syndromes." Due to the complexity of retinal degenerations, a retinal specialist will likely be involved in the diagnosis and management of these conditions.

Symptoms: What You May Experience • The first symptom that is usually noticed in RP is difficulty seeing in dim light. Patches or rings of blurred or darkened vision, termed "scotomas," may develop. These typically affect far or mid-peripheral vision first and progress to involve more of the peripheral vision over time, leading to what is often referred to as "tunnel vision." Central vision is usually not affected until the late stages of the disease. In contrast, with CORD, you may first notice reduced central vision and difficulty with reading and sometimes, light aversion, or photophobia.

It is rare to lose all of your vision from an inherited retinal degeneration. However, legal blindness due to loss of peripheral vision is common in RP, and legal blindness due to decreased central vision (less than 20/200) may occur in CORD or other macular dystrophies.

Examination Findings: What the Doctor Looks For • The eye doctor will examine the back of the eye looking for changes in the retina that are characteristic of RP, CORD, or macular dystrophy. In the early stages, the retina may look relatively normal. Later, dark pigmented deposits tend to develop in the retina. The optic nerve may also look pale, retinal blood vessels can become narrowed, and cataracts may develop within the first three or four decades of life. Swelling of the retina, called cystoid macular edema, may also develop in patients with RP.

The eye doctor will need to perform tests to confirm the diagnosis and monitor the course of the disease. A typical test is a visual field test, which maps the quality of your central and peripheral vision. An electroretinogram or an electrooculography may be done; these are non-invasive tests that help determine the health of the eye by measuring retinal electrical signals in dark and light conditions. Lastly, molecular genetic testing may be performed. There are nearly 350 different genetic causes of RP and the many inherited retinal degenerations that are related to it.

What You Can Do • While there is currently no treatment to stop or prevent the development of an inherited retinal degeneration, regular followup with your eye doctor is important for monitoring the condition and optimizing visual function.

When to Call the Doctor • You should see your eye doctor as soon as you notice changes in your central or peripheral vision, if you have persistent difficulty seeing in dim light, or if you develop increased sensitivity to light. It is important to have regular followups with an ophthalmologist and, whenever possible, with a retinal degeneration specialist in order to undergo molecular genetic testing, monitor for complications, and receive treatment if appropriate.

Treatment • There is nothing yet available to completely prevent or stop the development of RP or other inherited retinal degenerations. However, many trials have shown that supplementation regimens with different vitamins and other nutrients are helpful in delaying the progression of RP. Use of these supplements can prolong useful vision and buy additional time until gene therapy and other treatment options become available. It is important to note that certain supplements are not recommended and can even be harmful in certain types of inherited retinal degenerations,

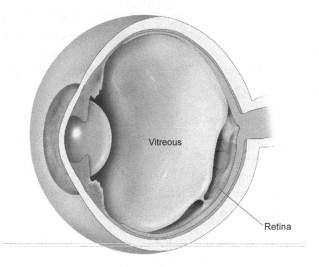

11.3. The vitreous gel separates from the retina in a posterior vitreous detachment.

so only use supplements recommended to you by your eye doctor. Complications such as cystoid macular edema and cataracts can be treated if they develop to improve vision.

The FDA has already approved one type of gene therapy, and other such approaches are likely to be approved in the near future. With ongoing research, we are learning more about the genetic causes and underlying disease mechanisms of retinal dystrophies. This allows eye doctors to implement and develop far better and more specific treatment approaches.

One exciting new treatment option for advanced RP is the surgically implanted Argus II artificial retinal device, which has already been approved by the FDA and is available for patients with end-stage disease. Your eye doctor can also keep abreast of new clinical trials and treatment options.

Low vision and occupational therapy specialists can help you function at your highest possible level despite having decreased vision and help you achieve partial visual rehabilitation. There are also patient-driven organizations and support groups to help you cope with the symptoms.

Those affected with more complex syndromes usually need a team of doctors to help manage the other health issues. Additionally, certain dietary supplements may require periodic monitoring in the form of blood tests performed by your primary care doctor. For example, if you are taking vitamin A, then liver-function monitoring may be needed every year or so, and bone-density checks are needed in women with osteoporosis while on this supplement.

Prognosis: Will I See Better? • In general, RP and other hereditary retinal degenerations cause progressively worsening vision over years. However, most people with inherited retinal degenerations maintain useful central or peripheral vision well into middle age or longer. Vision can improve if complications are managed successfully and promptly, and if a restorative treatment strategy is implemented.

Additional Resource

https://eyewiki.aao.org/Retinitis_Pigmentosa

Color Blindness

BRIAN STAGG, MD AND PRATAP CHALLA, MD

What Is It? • Color blindness is a deficiency in the way colors are seen. With this condition, a person has difficulty distinguishing certain colors, such as red and green or blue and yellow. Red-green color deficiency is by far the most common form of color blindness; blue-yellow color deficiency is less common. The cone cells of the retina are responsible for allowing us to see color. Each cone contains a specific pigment— either red, green, or blue. Color blindness occurs when one of these color pigments is missing or defective. The deficiency may be partial (affecting only some shades of a color) or complete (affecting all shades of the color). Usually people with color vision problems are born with them. Color blindness affects more men than women, because of the way the defective gene is inherited. Approximately 1 in 12 men has at least some color perception problems. It is extremely rare not to be able to distinguish any color at all—this condition is called achromatopsia and is usually accompanied by other serious eye problems.

Some other diseases that can lead to color blindness include retinitis pigmentosa, optic neuropathy, Alzheimer's disease, diabetes mellitus, glaucoma, leukemia, liver disease, chronic alcoholism, age-related macular degeneration, multiple sclerosis, Parkinson's disease, and sickle-cell anemia. Injuries or strokes that damage the retina, optic nerve, or particular areas of the brain can also lead to color blindness. Some medications, such as certain antibiotics, barbiturates, anti-tuberculosis drugs, high blood pressure medications, and several medications used to treat autoimmune and psychiatric problems, can cause color vision changes as well.

Symptoms: What You May Experience • Certain colors may appear gray, or two colors that appear different to people without color blindness may appear similar to a person with color blindness. People who are born with color vision problems may not notice the difficulty that they have in distinguishing certain colors when they are young.

Examination Findings: What the Doctor Looks For • The eye doctor will perform a color vision test, of which several types are available, to determine if color blindness is present. Some color tests ask you to distinguish a colored figure or number from a background, while other tests involve identifying and grouping similar colors together.

What You Can Do • There is no known prevention for color blindness. Because the disease is often inherited, tell your eye doctor if it is present in your family. Your physician will recommend periodic vision exams if you are prescribed a medication that may cause color vision changes.

When to Call the Doctor • If you notice difficulty telling colors apart, call your eye doctor. A new color vision problem that was not present at birth may be a sign of another disease or a problem with a medication you are taking. Also, parents should be alert to symptoms of color blindness in their children.

Treatment • Inherited color blindness currently cannot be cured. Most people with color vision problems compensate well and rely on color cues and details or use adaptive equipment. Wearing glasses with tinted lenses can sometimes help those with achromatopsia who are also sensitive to bright light. Non-inherited color blindness that has a specific cause is treated by identifying and treating the underlying problem.

Prognosis: Will I See Better? • Inherited color blindness usually does not change over the course your lifetime. The prognosis for color blindness that occurs after birth depends on the underlying problem. For instance, if the color blindness is due to a medication, stopping the medication under a physician's guidance can often make color vision return to normal.

Additional Resources

https://www.preventblindness.org/color-blindness
https://www.aao.org/eye-health/diseases/what-is-color-blindness

Laser Treatment of Retinal Diseases

ANANTH SASTRY, MD

A variety of retinal diseases can be treated in the office with specialized laser procedures. Laser treatment may be performed the same day as your scheduled eye exam and does not require preoperative fasting.

What Can I Expect for Laser Retinal Surgery? • During your clinic visit, your eye doctor will bring you to a special laser room to perform the procedure. Your eye will first be numbed with an eye drop or an injection around the eye. Then your eye doctor may place a specialized contact lens on your eye as you sit with your chin in the chin rest of the laser delivery machine. Alternatively, your eye doctor may recline the procedure chair and perform the procedure with a head-mounted lighted laser. During the laser treatment, you may notice a bright flash of light and possibly a slight stinging sensation each time the laser fires. If this is bothersome, anesthetic eye drops or an injection may be given to ease the mild discomfort. The laser treatment is usually divided into two or more sessions on separate days. At the conclusion of the procedure, you may experience temporary blurred vision that resolves after several minutes or hours. Sometimes, you may bring a family member or a friend into the laser room during the procedure; however, they will need to wear protective laser goggles to prevent any potential damage to their eyes. There are several different types of retinal laser procedures that are used to treat different retinal conditions:

PANRETINAL LASER PHOTOCOAGULATION (PRP) Any disease that causes decreased oxygen to the retina, such as diabetic retinopathy or retinal vein occlusion, may cause the growth of abnormal new blood vessels in the eye, called neovascularization. Neovascularization in the back of the eye can lead to bleeding inside of the eye or a tractional

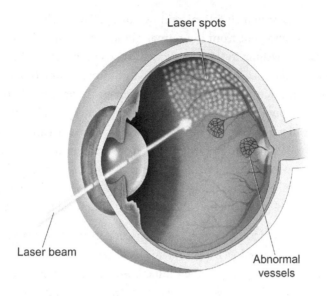

Laser spots

Laser beam

Abnormal
vessels

11.4. Laser surgery can slow the progression of diabetic
retinopathy.

retinal detachment, both of which can contribute to significantly decreased vision. Iris neovascularization can lead to neovascular glaucoma, which can cause severe pain and permanent vision loss from
uncontrolled high eye pressure. During PRP, laser is applied to the
peripheral retina in order to cause these abnormal blood vessels to
shrink. This lowers the probability of future bleeding or tractional retinal detachment. Thus, the goal of PRP is not to improve vision, but
rather to protect the eye from further harm.

Rarely, you may notice decreased vision in dim lighting, decreased side
vision, or blurry central vision caused by swelling of the retina after PRP
laser. Other rare side effects may include a spot in the central vision,
slight color vision or contrast abnormalities, a slight decrease in the ability to focus on near objects, or a larger pupil in the treated eye. These side
effects are generally less severe than the vision loss that might occur if the
neovascularization were left untreated.

FOCAL LASER FOR MACULAR EDEMA Focal laser is performed for
swelling in the macula, or central retina, and is most commonly caused

by diabetes or branch retinal vein occlusion. The swelling occurs due to fluid leaking out from the retinal blood vessels into the surrounding tissue. Swelling in the central retina can cause distorted or blurred vision. Additionally, if the swelling is left untreated for a prolonged period of time, it may cause permanent damage to the retina in the same way that a pool of water may damage a wooden floor if left alone for a prolonged period of time. The purpose of focal laser treatment is not to improve vision but to prevent vision from worsening; however vision may improve after treatment. Even more rarely, vision could worsen after treatment or the patient could notice a spot in his/her central vision. There is usually no pain associated with focal laser treatment.

LASER RETINOPEXY Laser retinopexy is a non-invasive procedure that is used to treat a retinal break or some localized retinal detachments that are in the far periphery of the retina. Laser retinopexy is performed to prevent the retinal break or detachment from progressing further. The procedure works by placing laser spots around the retinal break to "tack down" the surrounding retina. The scars formed by the laser take about one week to form, and thus the laser retinopexy does not produce an immediate effect. Laser retinopexy does not get rid of the floaters that you may have noticed as a result of your retinal break. Since the laser retinopexy does not have an immediate effect, it is important to recognize the symptoms of retinal detachment even after the laser treatment. These may include flashing lights, new floaters, or a visual field defect (often described as a dark curtain or shade coming across your field of view from any direction). If you notice these symptoms, you should return to your eye doctor immediately. Progression to a retinal detachment often requires surgical intervention in the operating room to repair.

PHOTODYNAMIC THERAPY FOR CHOROIDAL NEOVASCULARIZATION For certain types of choroidal neovascularization (CNV) affecting the center of the macula, photodynamic therapy (PDT) may be indicated. This treatment involves a light-activated intravenous dye (verteporfin) that is administered through a vein in your arm over 10 minutes. Five minutes after the dye has finished infusing, the laser light is applied to the CNV where the dye has collected. The special dye and light prevent damage to the normal surrounding retina. Several PDT treatments over several years may be needed to treat the CNV completely.

One rare potential side effect of the verteporfin dye is the temporary development of lower back pain. The cause of this lower back pain is unknown and affects roughly 2% of patients, but only while the dye is being administered. Additionally, you must avoid direct sunlight for roughly 5 days after the procedure to prevent burns on your skin and damage to your eyes.

SUBTHRESHOLD MICROPULSE LASER TREATMENT A newer form of laser treatment is now available for certain retinal diseases such as diabetic macular edema, macular edema from retinal vein occlusion, and central serous chorioretinopathy. With this procedure, laser spots are applied to the macula (the portion of the retina responsible for central vision) in a very gentle manner to cause microscopic changes in the cells of the retina without damaging those cells. The procedure is performed in a similar manner to the focal laser procedure described above. While this procedure involves less risk of retinal damage compared to focal laser treatment, it may not be as effective and may require another laser procedure or other treatment if it fails.

Additional Resources

https://eyewiki.aao.org/Lasers_(surgery)

https://eyewiki.aao.org/Panretinal_Photocoagulation

https://eyewiki.aao.org/Sub-threshold_Laser

https://eyewiki.aao.org/Photodynamic_Therapy_(PDT)

Retinal Surgery

VINCENT A. DERAMO, MD

Eye surgery has made great advances in recent years. Today, there are numerous eye conditions and diseases that can benefit from surgery. Many eye surgeries, such as cataract surgery and corneal transplantation, involve the front portion of the eye. Retinal surgery is performed on the back part of the eye. Only your eye doctor can determine whether you would benefit from retinal surgery. In general, there are two basic types of retinal surgery: vitrectomy and scleral buckling.

VITRECTOMY The back of the eye contains a gel-like material called vitreous, which makes up over 80% of the eye's volume. Surgical removal of the vitreous gel is called vitrectomy. The vitreous is not needed to see well and can safely be removed when necessary. The vitreous gel is involved in many retinal disorders, such as diabetic retinopathy, retinal detachment, macular hole, and epiretinal membrane, among others, and as such, vitrectomy surgery may benefit some eyes with these conditions.

As with any medical procedure, there are risks (1%) associated with vitrectomy which your surgeon will review with you. The surgery is performed in an operating room with either local or general anesthesia. Under local anesthesia, you will be awake but sedated, and a numbing medicine will be placed around your surgical eye. You will not see the surgery. Most patients find this comfortable without any significant pain during the procedure. In other cases, especially in younger patients, general anesthesia is used so that you may sleep through the procedure.

Vitrectomy is performed using a surgical microscope. The surgical eye is dilated so that the retina can be visualized by the surgeon. After the eye is cleaned with a sterilizing soap solution, three very small incisions are made in the sclera (the white outer layer of the eyeball). An infusion line is placed through one of these incisions to allow a balanced salt solution to flow into the eye and replace the vitreous gel during surgery. Very small, specialized instruments are used to remove the vitreous gel without harming the retina. Often other retinal procedures, such as laser treatment, membrane peeling (removal of scar tissue), removal of retained cataract material, retinal reattachment, and administration of certain medications into the vitreous cavity, are performed in combination with vitrectomy.

At the end of vitrectomy, it is sometimes necessary to place an air or gas bubble in the vitreous cavity. This bubble helps to hold the retina in place while it heals. Depending on the type of gas used, the bubble will last from a few days to many weeks before it dissolves completely on its own. While the bubble is present, the surgeon may ask you to hold your head in a certain position, such as face down or right or left side down. It is very important to avoid flying in an airplane, traveling to very high altitudes, or receiving nitrous oxide anesthesia when you have a bubble in your eye, since these may cause the bubble to expand and injure the eye. Also, you should alert other doctors if you require surgery elsewhere on the body when you have a gas bubble in the eye. If silicone oil is used to fill the vitreous cavity instead of gas, you can fly in an airplane, go to

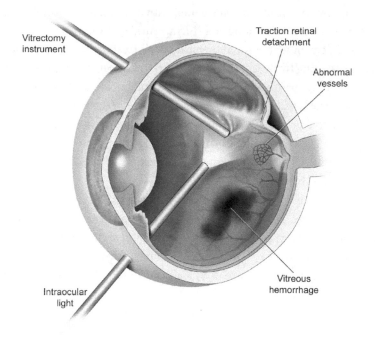

Vitrectomy
instrument

Traction retinal
detachment

Abnormal
vessels

Intraocular
light

Vitreous
hemorrhage

11.5. Instruments placed in eyeball for vitrectomy surgery.

high altitudes, and receive nitrous oxide anesthesia. However, silicone oil does not dissolve or disappear on its own as gas does, so it may need to be removed in a second operation at a later date,

After vitrectomy, the eye may be red and feel "scratchy" or irritated for a few days. The surgeon will prescribe eye drops for use after surgery. Typically, the eye is reexamined the day after surgery and then periodically. Complete healing can take up to a year.

SCLERAL BUCKLING In scleral buckling, a permanent solid silicone, nonmagnetic band called a buckle is placed around the eyeball, like a belt, to support the retina. Buckles have been safely used for many years and are well tolerated by the eye. Unlike vitrectomy, which is used to treat several retinal disorders, scleral buckling is mainly used to repair a retinal detachment. There are risks (1%) associated with scleral buckling surgery that your surgeon will discuss with you. The surgery is performed in an operating room, with either local or general anesthesia.

During surgery, the eye is first cleaned with a sterilizing soap solution. Your surgeon examines the retina during surgery to locate the retinal breaks and detachment. Retinal breaks may be treated with cryotherapy, which is a freezing treatment that helps the retina to remain in proper position, or with laser treatment. Then, the scleral buckle is placed around the eyeball. The buckle itself is a permanent piece of flexible material, often solid silicone or rarely, silicone sponge. The buckle is secured to the sclera underneath the conjunctiva, supporting the retina and repairing the detachment. The buckle is not visible after surgery, as it is placed far back on the eye, behind the eyelids.

Sometimes, as in vitrectomy, an air or gas bubble is used in scleral buckling, and the surgeon may ask you to hold your head in a certain position, such as face down or right or left side down. The eye may be red and feel irritated or "scratchy" for up to a few weeks after surgery. You will use eye drops after surgery, and the eye is typically reexamined the day after surgery, then periodically.

If you are undergoing retinal surgery, you will likely have further questions which should be discussed with your surgeon. In many cases, retinal surgery is extremely valuable in restoring vision lost as a result of severe retinal diseases that were untreatable in the not-so-distant past.

Additional Resources

https://www.aao.org/eye-health/diseases/what-is-vitrectomy
https://www.healthline.com/health/scleral-buckling

12 · Infection and Inflammation of the Eye

Uveitis

PRITHVI MRUTHYUNJAYA, MD, MHS

What Is It? • Uveitis means inflammation of the uveal tract, which is the pigmented portion of the eyeball composed of the iris, ciliary body, and choroid. These structures have an abundant blood supply, which makes them susceptible to inflammation and infections from other parts of the body. Our individual immune systems play an important role in determining the development and severity of the inflammation, so episodes of uveitis will be different in each person.

The most common classification of uveitis is based on the structures of the eye that are inflamed. Anterior uveitis (also called iritis or iridocyclitis) is inflammation in the front of the eye, in the anterior chamber and iris; intermediate uveitis (also called pars planitis) is inflammation in the front and middle part of the eye, in the anterior chamber, iris, and part of the vitreous cavity; posterior uveitis involves the back part of the eye in the retina and vitreous; and panuveitis involves all structures, from the front to the back of the eyeball.

Uveitis may be caused or made worse by an eye injury or various systemic illnesses, including infections and autoimmune diseases (when the body's immune system begins to attack its own uveal tract). Often, a specific cause cannot be identified despite a careful medical examination and laboratory testing. Your doctor will still try to determine the exact reason why the uveitis occurred so that they will be able to treat the underlying cause as well as the inflammation itself.

Symptoms: What You May Experience • You may experience eye pain, redness, light sensitivity, and blurry vision. In posterior uveitis and panuveitis, there is a greater chance of having decreased vision, because the choroid toward the back of the eye is affected.

Examination Findings: What the Doctor Looks For • Your eye doctor will ask about your medical history. Because all parts of the eye can be affected, a complete dilated eye exam is performed to assess the degree of inflammation in different parts of the eye. Your eye doctor will look specifically for inflammatory cells floating in your eyeball. The eye pressure is measured, since uveitis can sometimes lead to glaucoma. Additional imaging, including fluorescein angiography and ultrasound, may be performed. In some cases, your doctor may order laboratory tests to help identify the underlying cause. An evaluation by your primary medical doctor may also be required. In very severe cases, a sample of eye fluid may be removed with vitrectomy surgery and tested to determine the exact cause of the inflammation.

What You Can Do • Avoiding eye injury helps to prevent uveitis. If you have an underlying systemic autoimmune disease, controlling it with the help of your primary medical doctor may help to prevent uveitis in the future.

When to Call the Doctor • If you develop eye pain and redness, blurry vision, or new light sensitivity, you should contact your eye doctor.

Treatment • Typically your eye doctor will begin treatment with frequent steroid eye drops (up to once every hour while awake), which will be gradually used less often over weeks to months. Sometimes severe inflammation (usually in posterior uveitis or panuveitis) may require oral steroids or steroid injections around the eyeball. Your doctor will monitor you for any harmful eye and systemic side effects that can be caused by steroid medications (such as cataract and glaucoma). In the most severe cases, oral or injected immunosuppressive medicines are prescribed, typically with the assistance of your primary medical doctor or rheumatologist. Your doctor will treat any other infections or illnesses that may be related to your uveitis.

Prognosis: Will I See Better? • Uveitis can be a long-standing, recurrent inflammatory condition. The severity and extent of the inflammation will determine the extent of improvement. Prompt diagnosis and treatment with steroids will often restore vision to good levels. If you have uveitis, follow your doctor's instructions about your prescribed medications and report any changes in your vision promptly.

Additional Resources

https://www.aao.org/eye-health/diseases/what-is-uveitis
https://eyewiki.aao.org/Acute_Anterior_Uveitis
https://eyewiki.aao.org/Treatment_of_Uveitis

Endophthalmitis

HENRY L. FENG, MD

What Is It? • Endophthalmitis is a serious inflammatory reaction inside the eyeball, most often due to a bacterial, fungal, or viral infection. Microbes may enter the eye after trauma, eye surgery, or an eye injection (exogenous endophthalmitis), or may spread to the eye through the bloodstream from other parts of the body (endogenous endophthalmitis). Endophthalmitis after cataract or other eye surgery most often occurs within 2–7 days; however, it can also occur months or years later in certain cases, especially after glaucoma surgery.

Symptoms: What You May Experience • Symptoms may include decreased vision, eye pain, eye redness, and eye discharge. These symptoms may develop rapidly in some cases.

Examination Findings: What the Doctor Looks For • Your eye doctor will perform a complete eye exam, which includes checking your vision, eye pressure, pupil reaction to light, and dilating your pupil so that they can look for signs of infection inside your eye. In some cases, an ultrasound of the eyeball may be performed.

What You Can Do • There is no proven method for preventing endophthalmitis; however, you can reduce the spread of germs by practicing good hygiene. This includes washing your hands with clean soap and water before touching your face or eyes and keeping the tips of your eye drop bottles clean. These practices are particularly important to follow after an eye surgery or eye injection.

When to Call the Doctor • If you develop new, severe eye pain, redness, discharge, or loss of vision after eye surgery, contact your eye surgeon the same day or go to an emergency room and ask to be seen by an eye doctor as soon as possible. Prompt diagnosis and treatment of endophthalmitis is crucial to minimize the chance of significant vision loss.

Treatment • Endophthalmitis may be treated by injecting antibiotics directly into the eye. This treatment can be performed in the office in most cases. Your doctor may remove a small sample of fluid from your eye for testing to find out if and what kind of infection is present and inject antibiotics into the eye. In more serious cases, you may need emergency vitrectomy surgery to remove the infection from the eye in addition to injection of antibiotics.

Prognosis: Will I See Better? • With prompt treatment, if you have mild endophthalmitis, you can recover excellent vision. Visual recovery can take weeks to months, and sometimes more than one antibiotic injection or surgery may be needed. In severe cases, vision may not improve, and rarely you may even lose the eye. The chance of visual improvement depends on the severity of the infection and how quickly it is treated.

Additional Resource

https://eyewiki.aao.org/Endophthalmitis

Viral Retinitis

PRITHVI MRUTHYUNJAYA, MD, MHS

What Is It? • A virus is an organism that lives by infecting other living cells. A virus can enter the human body through various routes—it can be inhaled in the air (as is influenza, or "flu"), ingested with food, or transmitted through contact with a living carrier of the virus. Once in the bloodstream, the virus can infect the body's cells and cause them to malfunction. However, viruses are usually attacked and controlled by the body's own immune system so that symptoms do not develop.

Viral retinitis is an extremely rare infection of the retina of one or both eyes caused by virus particles that enter the retina. Some forms of viral retinitis mainly affect those who have systemic illnesses that weaken their own immune systems, such as Acquired Immune Deficiency Syndrome (AIDS) or cancer. Certain medications such as steroids or chemotherapy can also weaken the immune system, increasing susceptibility to viral retinitis.

There are three viruses that are commonly responsible for viral retinitis: cytomegalovirus (CMV), varicella zoster virus (VZV—the virus that causes chicken pox), and herpes simplex virus (HSV— the virus that causes cold sores). Most people are exposed to CMV and VZV as children or young adults and then become immune to them, so these viruses typically only infect the retina in patients with weakened immune systems. HSV, a common cause of cold sores, can (rarely) infect the retina even in otherwise healthy patients—a condition called acute retinal necrosis syndrome.

Symptoms: What You May Experience • You may experience light sensitivity, floaters, and possibly flashing lights in one or both eyes. There may be a rapid decline in vision.

Examination Findings: What the Doctor Looks For • Your eye doctor will perform a full eye exam including a dilated exam to check for bleeding and/or whitening along the blood vessels of the normally clear retina. Your doctor may also need to push on the eye to look for a retinal tear or detachment.

What You Can Do • There is nothing that can be done to prevent viral retinitis itself. Because AIDS patients are more at risk for developing viral retinitis, preventing the spread of HIV is especially important. HIV-positive patients with CD4 counts of < 50 need regular eye exams to check for early viral retinitis.

When to Call the Doctor • If you develop blurry vision and sensitivity to light, especially if you have a weakened immune system, you should call your eye doctor promptly.

Treatment • Your eye doctor will determine if you have an underlying health condition that might predispose you to the development of viral retinitis, and if so, they will refer you to your primary medical doctor for additional treatment. The retinal infection is usually treated for several weeks with a combination of oral, intravenous, and intraocular antiviral medications (such as ganciclovir, acyclovir, or foscarnet), depending on which virus is suspected to be the cause. In cases of CMV retinitis, an effective surgical procedure involves inserting a long-lasting pellet of ganciclovir into the vitreous gel to directly treat the retinal infection.

Prognosis: Will I See Better? • Although the medications used to treat viral retinitis are getting better, the improvement in vision that can be achieved once the infection is controlled depends on the severity of retinal damage caused by the virus as well as how early the infection is diagnosed and how soon it is treated.

Additional Resources

https://eyewiki.aao.org/CMV_Retinitis
https://eyewiki.aao.org/Acute_retinal_necrosis

13 · Tumors of the Eye and Orbit

Retinoblastoma

ANN SHUE, MD

What Is It? • Retinoblastoma is a serious cancer that develops inside the eye and primarily affects children. It is usually a white or cream-colored growth that starts from the inner lining of the eye wall, called the retina, and can grow to fill the eyeball and/or spread to other organs. Treatment goals include first, saving the patient's life and second, keeping as much sight as possible. Retinoblastoma is rare and affects only about 4 children in every 1 million under the age of 15 years in the United States. It makes up about 3% of all cancers in children <15 years old. About 2/3 are diagnosed before they are 2 years old. It may be present in both eyes at the same time, especially if diagnosed in the first year of life.

What Causes It? • While a baby is in the womb, embryonic retinal cells or immature retina cells multiply to create the retina. Normally, these embryonic retinal cells eventually stop multiplying and just mature. There is a gene that we all have, called the RB1 gene, that works to control our body's cells from overreplicating. When this gene mutates so it cannot work anymore, the body loses control of some cells. With no control from a mutated RB1 gene, the embryonic retinal cells continue to multiply with no stopping point. In about 25–30% of patients, the gene mutation is present in all cells of their body (germline mutation, heritable form) because they inherited it from a parent or the mutation happened early in gestation by chance (most heritable forms are due to a random mutation early in development). In 70–75%, only a single cell develops the mutated gene (nonheritable form) by chance, which then begins to divide to form a tumor. Scientists do not yet know exactly what triggers these random mutations.

Examination Findings: What the Doctor Looks For • The eye doctor (usually a pediatric ophthalmologist or retina specialist) will perform a complete eye exam with dilation to look in the back of the eye for any abnormal growths or masses. Ultrasound may also be used to look for masses or for characteristics such as calcification, which may be associated with retinoblastoma. If the child is too young to cooperate with the exam, an examination under anesthesia (EUA) may be needed. A radiographic scan of the head may also be ordered to look at the eyes, eye socket, and brain. Magnetic resonance imaging (MRI) is the recommended type of imaging.

When to Call the Doctor • A white pupillary reflex (leukocoria, often noticed on a photo with flash), crossing or drifting eyes (strabismus), decreased vision, red and painful eye, one pupil larger than the other, or any change someone can see in the front of the eye or in the position of the eye should prompt a visit to the eye doctor for a full, dilated eye exam.

Treatment • To provide the best possible treatment, many types of professionals need to be involved, and caregivers, usually parents, are a crucial part of the team. There are centers of excellence for retinoblastoma around the world (http://www.1rbw.org) where, if possible, evaluation is recommended before treatment begins. The treatment plan depends on whether one or both eyes are affected, how many retinoblastoma lesions there are, how big they are, and where they are located. A lesion alone cannot be taken out of the eye without danger of spreading the tumor. Sometimes, the best way to remove the lesion and cure retinoblastoma is to remove the whole eye and replace it with a prosthesis. Other times, chemotherapy (whole body or through the blood supply that serves the eye) can be given to shrink retinoblastoma lesions and then any remaining lesion can be lasered or frozen (cryotherapy). Radiation is also an option; however, it can increase the risk of new tumors forming later in the child's life. Newer radiation techniques, such as proton-beam radiation, are more precise and may reduce the risk of secondary tumor development. Radiation may also be focused onto a lesion with a plate that is placed directly over the mass (plaque brachytherapy).

Prognosis: What Are the Survival Rates? • With more advanced ways to diagnose and treat retinoblastoma, the prognosis has significantly improved. When looking at the 3-year mark after treatment, about 96% of patients who had retinoblastoma in one or both eyes are alive. However, survivors are prone to developing another cancer later in life, such as bone, blood, lung, or bladder cancer, which may be life threatening. In terms of vision, the prognosis is excellent in a case where only one eye is affected because the fellow eye is still normal. When both eyes are affected, the visual outcome depends on the size and location of the retinoblastoma lesion(s) upon diagnosis. The most important factors in improving the outcome are increased awareness, earlier recognition of the warning signs by family and doctors, and prompt diagnosis and treatment.

Additional Resources

https://eyewiki.aao.org/Retinoblastoma

https://www.cancer.org/cancer/retinoblastoma/about/what-is-retinoblastoma
    .html

Gallie, Brenda L., and Soliman, Sameh E. "Retinoblastoma." Taylor and Hoyt's
    Pediatric Ophthalmology and Strabismus. Ed. Scott R. Lambert and
    Christopher J Lyons. 5th ed. Edinburgh: Elsevier, 2017. Print.

Intraocular Melanoma

WAJIHA JURDI KHEIR, MD

What Is It? • Intraocular or uveal melanoma is a cancerous tumor that arises from the uveal coat of the eye (the pigmented tissues—the iris, ciliary body, and choroid). It is the most common primary (not spread from other parts of the body) intraocular tumor in adults and is frequently treated by an ocular oncologist (eye cancer specialist). Unlike skin melanoma, exposure to sunlight or other sources of ultraviolet light has not been linked to occurrence of intraocular melanoma. Northern European ancestry / Caucasian race, certain genetic factors, and family history have been associated with a higher incidence of choroidal melanoma.

There may also be benign choroidal pigmented lesions in the eye called nevi, similar to freckles or moles on the skin. These can be mistaken for melanoma but rarely turn into melanoma over time. Another benign pigmented lesion in the eye is a melanocytoma, which is deeply pigmented and arises very close to the optic nerve. It is often difficult to tell these different diseases apart, which is why consultation with a retina or ocular oncology specialist is important for making the right diagnosis.

Symptoms: What You May Experience • Uveal melanomas are usually asymptomatic until they grow large enough to disrupt vision. If the tumor originates from the iris or ciliary body, it may be detected on an un-dilated eye exam and sometimes can be seen while looking in a mirror. However, the more common choroidal type of melanoma can only be detected with a dilated eye exam by an eye doctor. If the tumor is close to the center of vision (macula) or optic nerve, or if it grows enough to leak fluid causing a retinal detachment, you may experience blurry vision, flashing lights, floaters, and dark areas in your visual field.

Examination Findings: What the Doctor Looks For • Your eye specialist will perform a thorough exam of the front and back portions of the eye, which includes a dilated eye exam to determine the location of the tumor, how close the tumor is to the optic nerve, whether it has certain features (drusen, orange pigment, fluid), and its diameter and thickness. You may also need to undergo several imaging studies such as fundus photos, autofluorescence, optical coherence tomography, fluorescein angiography, and ultrasonography.

What You Can Do • There is no proven way to prevent the development of an intraocular melanoma. Since melanomas often progress without any symptoms, you should be diligent in following up regularly with your eye doctor. If you have been told you have a freckle or nevus in the eye, make sure to always follow up with your doctor as instructed and have it photographed periodically to determine if it is growing.

When to Call the Doctor • If you experience new symptoms like blurry vision, floaters, flashing lights, or visual field defects, contact your eye doctor promptly.

Treatment • There are several options for treatment depending on the size of the tumor and the capabilities of the eye center and hospital. One possibility is enucleation or removing the eye, which is done when the tumor is too large or too thick to be safely treated locally. Eye-saving options for treatment include local radiation therapy or plaque brachytherapy, proton beam therapy, or external beam radiotherapy. Laser may be used in addition to radiation. Your ocular oncologist will also refer you to be screened for metastasis (spread of the tumor to other parts of the body). This screening will need to be performed on a regular basis for at least 10 years after a diagnosis of intraocular melanoma.

Prognosis: Will I See Better? • The priority in treating uveal melanoma is preserving life and preventing spread of the tumor, which is why continued screening for metastasis is needed. If an eye-saving treatment is chosen, the amount of remaining vision will depend on where the original tumor was located as well as what kind of radiation and how much radiation was given. Over time, the retina may become dysfunctional due to radiation therapy, resulting in possible retinal swelling or bleeding. These complications can be treated with laser to the retina as well as injections in and around the eye. Functional vision in the affected eye cannot be guaranteed.

Additional Resource

https://eyewiki.aao.org/Uveal_Melanoma

Other Tumors of the Retina and Choroid

WAJIHA JURDI KHEIR, MD

What Are They? • The most commonly diagnosed and treated intraocular tumors vary with age group. In children, the most common type of intraocular tumor originating from the eye is retinoblastoma. In adults, the most common type of intraocular tumor originating from the eye is uveal melanoma. In this section, other tumors of the retina and choroid are described.

RETINAL TUMORS There are several categories of retinal tumors. Vascular tumors such as retinal hemangioblastomas are benign but can cause complications from bleeding or leaking fluid under the retina. They can be associated with a hereditary disease called von Hippel–Lindau (VHL). Acquired vascular (vasoproliferative) tumors usually occur in older individuals with high blood pressure, are benign, and are treated when complications such as bleeding or retinal detachment occur.

Other tumors can arise from the neural and neural-supporting cells. Astrocytic hamartomas are benign tumors that usually occur in childhood and are associated with a condition called tuberous sclerosis. They are usually stable but may occasionally exhibit rapid growth and cause retinal detachment or glaucoma. Acquired astrocytomas, while still benign, occur in adulthood and are commonly progressive and disruptive.

Tumors can also arise from the layer of cells between the retina and the choroid known as the retinal pigment epithelium. Congenital hypertrophy of retinal pigment epithelium (CHRPE) is a benign growth of these cells. Tumors called adenomas (benign) and adenocarcinomas (malignant) can also arise from these cells but are exceedingly rare.

Lymphoma can occur in the retina and vitreous gel and is frequently associated with a central nervous system lymphoma. Vision may be blurred due to lymphoid cells collecting in the vitreous and underneath the retina.

CHOROIDAL TUMORS The choroid is the part of the uveal tract located between the retina and sclera. Choroidal hemangiomas are benign vascular tumors that usually occur close to the optic nerve and macula and can cause visual disturbances if fluid leaks under the retina. Choroidal osteomas are benign growths of bone tissue that usually occur in young adult women and may be associated with the growth of abnormal leaky blood vessels that can lead to blurring of vision. Lymph tissue may also grow within the choroid and is called benign lymphoid hyperplasia; this can be difficult to distinguish from uveal malignant lymphoma, which is often associated with lymphoma in other parts of the body.

METASTATIC TUMORS Metastatic cancerous tumors from other parts of the body are the most common eye tumors found in adults. These cancer cells spread through the bloodstream to the choroid and retina. Breast and lung cancer are the most common types of cancer that spread to the eye. Metastases can affect one eye in multiple areas or can affect both eyes. In some people, a metastatic tumor in the eye is the first identifiable sign of cancer. Systemic lymphoma can often lead to ocular involvement and affect the choroid as mentioned above.

What You Can Do • Be proactive about your health since the most common overall tumor affecting the eye is spread from cancer located in other parts of the body. Maintain regular primary care appointments, perform recommended screening tests, and have a yearly, dilated eye exam.

When to Call the Doctor • If you develop blurry vision, floaters, flashes, or dark areas in your visual field, you should contact your eye doctor promptly.

Treatment • Available treatments for tumors of the retina and choroid vary widely. Depending on the type, size, and location of the tumor, appropriate treatments may range from careful periodic monitoring to laser, freezing treatments, radiation, chemotherapy, injections in the eye, or even surgery. Your eye doctor will help you decide the appropriate treatment for your particular situation. If the tumor in the eye has spread (metastasized) to the eye from another part of the body, your oncologist will also be actively involved in the treatment plan.

Prognosis: Will I See Better? • With most benign tumors, the treatment goal is to improve or preserve vision. If the tumor is located in areas of the retina or choroid responsible for central vision, vision may be limited after treatment. However, advances in treatment options have enabled eye doctors to maintain functional vision in many patients.

Additional Resources

https://cycwiki.aao.org/Intraocular_Vascular_Tumors

https://eyewiki.aao.org/Choroidal_Osteoma

https://www.aao.org/eyenet/article/retinal-astrocytoma

Tumors of the Orbit

ROSHNI RANJIT-REEVES, MD

What Is the Orbit? • The orbit is a bony cavity in the skull in which the eye and a surrounding complex of tissues are situated. It is pear-shaped and about 30 milliliters in volume. It is composed of seven bones and provides protection for the eye, blood vessels, periorbital muscles (muscles of the eyelid), extraocular muscles (muscles on the eye), nerves, lymphatics, fatty tissue, cranial nerves, lacrimal gland, and tear duct system. Any of these structures can grow abnormally and form tumors.

Which Tumors Involve the Orbit? • Tumors of the orbit can be either benign or malignant (cancerous). Common benign orbital tumors include hemangiomas (tumors of the blood vessels), lymphangiomas (tumors of lymphatics), lipomas (tumors of fat cells), and neurofibromas and schwannomas (tumors of nerve tissue). However, these cell types can also grow to form malignant tumors in some patients. Angiosarcomas and hemangiopericytomas are malignant blood-vessel tumors and liposarcomas are malignant tumors of fatty tissue. Malignant peripheral nerve sheath tumors can arise from originally benign neurofibromas in patients with diseases such as neurofibromatosis. Lymphomas also can occur in the orbit because of the lymphatic tissues normally present in the orbit. The lacrimal gland, which produces tears, can give rise to tumors in the lateral portion of the orbit. They are usually benign in nature (such as a pleomorphic adenoma), but can be very aggressive and malignant (such as adenoid cystic carcinoma which can spread to surrounding areas and along the nerves).

Malignant tumors of the orbit also include malignant tumors of muscle and meninges (the tissue sheath that covers the optic nerve and the brain). Rhabdomyosarcoma is a malignant tumor that most commonly forms from the skeletal (voluntary) muscle cells in children, while leiomyosarcoma is a malignant tumor of smooth (involuntary) muscle cells more commonly in adults. Orbital meningiomas are benign tumors of the meninges, which is the protective covering around the brain and optic nerve. These tumors can wrap around the optic nerve and travel back into the brain.

Tumors within the eye can grow outward into the orbit and can also spread to the brain. Tumors in the brain can also grow toward the orbit and affect the eye. Tumors of the orbit can affect vision by compressing the optic nerve and surrounding nerves and muscles, which can then affect the muscles of the eyeball, sometimes resulting in double vision.

In adults, the spread of cancer cells from other parts of the body (metastasis) to the orbit is also possible. These metastatic tumors to the orbit can even be the first presenting sign of cancer located in other parts of the body. The most common metastatic tumors to the orbit are from lung or breast cancer, but they can spread from nearly any other site.

Additional Resources

https://eyewiki.aao.org/Orbital_masses

http://www.eyecancer.com/

http://www.eyecancerinfo.com

14 · The Optic Nerve

Optic Neuropathy

JAMES H. POWERS, MD

What Is It? • Optic neuropathy is broadly defined as any disease, condition, or abnormal functioning of the optic nerve, which is the structure that connects the eye to the brain. The optic nerve carries visual information from the eye to the brain, where it is processed to help form the images that we see.

There are many possible causes of optic neuropathy, including poor blood flow, inflammation, infection, inherited diseases, tumors compressing the optic nerve, glaucoma, trauma, toxins, nutritional deficiencies, and radiation. The most common cause of optic neuropathy in younger adults is optic neuritis, which is an inflammation of the optic nerve; in older adults, the most common cause is ischemic optic neuropathy which is a decrease in blood supply to the optic nerve.

Symptoms: What You May Experience • The most common symptom of optic neuropathy is trouble with vision in one eye, which may manifest as blurred vision, a "film" over your vision, difficulty distinguishing colors, or dark areas in your visual field. Eye pain may also be present depending on the cause. The vision changes and eye pain may develop rapidly or may progress over weeks to months. Rarely, both eyes may be affected. You should report any other symptoms you may be experiencing, even in other parts of your body, to your eye doctor so that they may best determine the cause of your optic neuropathy.

Examination Findings: What the Doctor Looks For • Your eye doctor will check your level of vision, peripheral vision, pupils, and eye pressure. They will also dilate your eyes to visualize your optic nerve and check for any evidence of swelling or pallor. The doctor may also order brain imaging, most commonly magnetic resonance imaging (MRI), to assess the health of the brain, optic nerve, and structures surrounding your eyes. In some cases, blood tests, a lumbar puncture (also known as a spinal tap, which allows analysis of the fluid that surrounds your brain, spinal cord, and optic nerve), and other specialized tests may be performed to determine the underlying cause of your optic neuropathy.

What You Can Do • Only some causes of optic neuropathy can be prevented. To help prevent traumatic optic neuropathy, wear eye protection to avoid eye injury. To help prevent optic neuropathy caused by poor blood flow, take care of your general health including your cholesterol level, blood pressure, and blood sugar levels if you are diabetic. To help prevent nutritional and toxic optic neuropathies, avoid excessive alcohol intake, smoking, or other toxic exposures.

When to Call the Doctor • If you begin to experience partial vision loss or blurriness, difficulty distinguishing colors, eye pain, or any other changes to your vision, you should call your eye doctor. Prompt medical attention is the best way to ensure optimal outcomes.

Treatment • There is no way to completely reverse an optic neuropathy once it has occurred. Treatment of an optic neuropathy will depend on the specific cause and may lead to some improvement. If you have had an optic neuropathy caused by blood-flow problems in one eye, taking blood-thinning medications such as aspirin may help protect against a similar optic neuropathy in the second eye. Controlling your cholesterol, blood sugar, and blood pressure through medications, diet, and exercise may also be helpful. Your eye doctor may choose to treat optic neuropathy caused by inflammation or injury with anti-inflammatory or steroid medications. If your optic neuropathy is caused by a bacterial infection, antibiotic treatment would be needed. Optic neuropathy caused by glaucoma may be treated with medications that lower eye pressure. If a tumor is compressing the optic nerve causing optic neuropathy, medical and surgical treatment to reduce tumor size may be required.

Prognosis: Will I See Better? • Certain optic neuropathies may be successfully treated, while others may be difficult or impossible to treat. Visual outcomes depend on the cause, severity, and duration of the optic neuropathy. Once damage has occurred to the optic nerve, it is difficult to reverse. Treatment in those circumstances is aimed at preventing future vision loss or occurrence of a similar optic neuropathy in the other eye.

Additional Resources

https://eyewiki.aao.org/Optic_Atrophy

https://www.aao.org/eye-health/diseases/what-is-ischemic-optic-neuropathy

Glaucoma

MICHAEL S. QUIST, MD AND CLAUDIA S. COHEN, MD

What Is It? • Glaucoma is one of the leading cause of blindness in the United States and the second leading cause of blindness around the world. It is progressive and insidious in onset: often a person with glaucoma will be completely unaware of the condition until it is quite advanced. If glaucoma is detected early enough, it can be treated.

Glaucoma is 4- to 6-times more common in those who are black, but people of all ethnic backgrounds are at risk. Family history is a significant risk factor. Tell your eye doctor if anyone in your family has had glaucoma or even potential glaucoma (glaucoma suspect). Glaucoma has traditionally been associated with high eye pressure. It is possible, however, to have normal eye pressure and still have glaucoma.

Symptoms: What You May Experience • Glaucoma is actually an umbrella term that includes a group of diseases that damage the optic nerve. Primary open angle glaucoma, the most common type, is typically asymptomatic at first, and therefore you may not realize that you have glaucoma until the vision has been significantly affected. This is because glaucoma progresses gradually, and typically affects peripheral vision before it affects central vision. Once you start to lose vision though, about 30–50% of the optic nerve has already been permanently damaged. There is no treatment that can restore vision once it is lost due to glaucoma. That is why prevention is key. There are some types of glaucoma that may be associated with eye pain, such as angle closure glaucoma. Usually the pain is rather significant and should be promptly evaluated by an eye doctor, preferably that same day.

Examination Findings: What the Doctor Looks For • Eye doctors are trained to look for signs of glaucoma before symptoms appear. An important part of the eye exam is measuring the eye pressure. The normal range for eye pressure is 9–21 mm Hg. Some people with glaucoma may

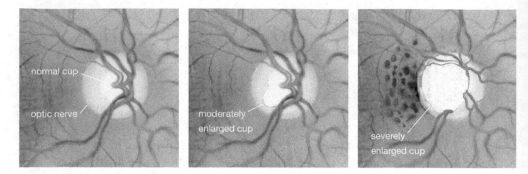

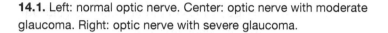

14.1. Left: normal optic nerve. Center: optic nerve with moderate glaucoma. Right: optic nerve with severe glaucoma.

have eye pressures above the normal range, while others may have glaucoma even with normal eye pressures (termed normal tension glaucoma).

If you do have high eye pressure, your eye doctor may measure the thickness of your cornea using an instrument called a pachymeter. Eyes with thicker corneas may also have higher measured eye pressures, whereas those with thinner corneas may have lower eye pressures. Thus, eye pressure and corneal thickness are used together to assess your risk for glaucoma and your long-term pressure goals. Both of these values can change with time, and eye pressure can also vary throughout the day. The cornea typically becomes thinner with age.

Your eye doctor will also perform a dilated eye exam to assess your optic nerve. If your eye doctor suspects that you may have glaucoma, they may take photographs or scans of your optic nerves as a basis for comparison during future exams. They may also ask you to perform a computerized visual field test to assess your peripheral vision. During this test, you sit in a dimly lit room and look into a large white bowl. You will be asked to look at a target straight ahead at the center of the bowl while you are shown a flashing light in your peripheral vision at the edge of the bowl. You will be asked to press a button each time you see the light. The test can be quite challenging and tiring, so you may be asked to come back at another time to repeat it.

What You Can Do • If you have glaucoma, you should use your eye drops as prescribed and follow up with your eye doctor regularly to prevent progression of glaucoma. Even if you do not have known glaucoma, it is still important to follow up regularly with an eye doctor. Because glaucoma is a slowly progressive disease, small changes may be apparent from year to year. There is a genetic component to glaucoma, so if you have a family member with the condition, you may be more likely to develop it.

When to Call the Doctor • Glaucoma is a disease that can take many years to develop. Because there are virtually no symptoms in the majority of cases, it is unlikely to require an emergency visit to your eye doctor. If you develop any changes in vision or suspect that you might have glaucoma, you should make an appointment with your eye doctor for a comprehensive eye exam. If you develop sudden, intense eye pain that lasts longer than several seconds, however, you should see your eye doctor right away, because certain types of glaucoma can cause pain.

Treatment • Once it has been determined that you have glaucoma, you will likely be started on an eye drop to lower your eye pressure. There are many types of eye drops available, and your doctor will choose the one that best suits you. Typically, you will be asked to return several weeks later to see how well the medicine is working. If it is working well, you are usually seen every few months to check for stability. If your eye pressure is still too high, other eye drops may be added, or treatments involving laser or surgery may be discussed.

Prognosis: Will I See Better? • Once glaucoma has damaged the optic nerve, those cells cannot regenerate. Visual outcome depends on the stage at which the disease was diagnosed, and prognosis varies greatly among patients. At this time, glaucoma treatment is aimed at preventing further vision loss; it does not restore vision already lost. Prevention is key.

Additional Resource

https://eyewiki.aao.org/Primary_Open-Angle_Glaucoma

Laser Treatment of Glaucoma

SUSAN M. WAKIL, MD

What Is It? • There are two different types of laser surgeries for glaucoma that your eye doctor may discuss with you. These laser procedures are performed in the office setting after numbing your eye with eye drops.

LASER PERIPHERAL IRIDOTOMY If the angle of your eye is crowded by the iris, then the eye is at risk for a sudden painful rise in eye pressure called acute angle closure glaucoma. To prevent this, a laser peripheral iridotomy is necessary. This procedure involves using a laser to create a little opening in your iris (colored portion of the eye) that allows an alternative pathway for the aqueous fluid to circulate within your eye.

SELECTIVE LASER TRABECULOPLASTY (SLT) This procedure can help lower the eye pressure. In turn, it may also help reduce the number or frequency of eye drops that you are using to lower the eye pressure. The SLT treatment stimulates the internal drainage system of your eye using low energy laser. This results in increased fluid drainage out of the eye and therefore lowers the eye pressure.

What You May Experience during the Procedure • Each of these procedures typically takes 10–15 minutes to perform. The laser procedure is performed using a machine that is similar to the slit lamp machine that your eye doctor uses to examine your eyes in a clinic. Thirty minutes prior to the laser procedure, your eye doctor may place an eye drop on the eye to help prevent a sudden increase in eye pressure after the laser treatment and may also place an eye drop to constrict your pupil. A numbing drop will be placed on your eye before starting, and a lens that touches the surface of your eye may be used to help magnify the part of the eye to be treated. There should be minimal pain, although you may feel some pressure or a small "pinch." It is important to remain still and follow the instructions of your eye doctor throughout the procedure.

Possible Complications • At the end of either procedure, your eye doctor may prescribe eye drops for a short period of time to minimize any inflammation from the laser procedure. Afterward, you may experience some temporary light sensitivity or a dull eye ache that will improve with time. Uncommonly, the pressure in the eye may rise temporarily after the procedure, and your eye doctor may administer eye drops or pills in the clinic. You should contact your eye doctor if you have persistent light sensitivity, eye pain, and/or a feeling of pressure in the eye.

Prognosis: Will I See Better? • The goal of these laser treatments is to lower your eye pressure, which may help prevent further vision loss from glaucoma in the future.

Additional Resources

https://eyewiki.aao.org/Laser_Peripheral_Iridotomy

https://www.aao.org/eye-health/diseases/glaucoma-treatment

Glaucoma Surgery

SUSAN M. WAKIL, MD

What Is It? • There is a range of surgeries that may be indicated at various disease stages based on the type of glaucoma and the severity.

MINIMALLY INVASIVE GLAUCOMA SURGERY (MIGS) MIGS is an umbrella term that includes a variety of procedures that target the angle of the eye, where fluid within the eye is internally drained. Some of these procedures are performed in combination with cataract surgery. These procedures are generally associated with fewer risks than the traditional glaucoma surgeries described here. However, this is counterbalanced by a more modest eye pressure reduction with MIGS procedures. Please see the next chapter for a more detailed description of the various MIGS procedures.

TRABECULECTOMY Trabeculectomy surgery is considered the most effective in lowering eye pressure, especially when very low pressures are needed to prevent worsening glaucoma or when other nonsurgical or less invasive techniques have failed. It involves the creation of a flap within the sclera (white covering of the eye) that will allow passage of the fluid from the inside of the eye to the outside of the eye to an area underneath the conjunctiva (clear tissue covering the white of the eye). During the surgery, certain medications are used to help keep the flap open and decrease scarring that may close the flap. Exiting fluid will create a "filtering bleb" or bubble underneath the conjunctiva, which will be located under the upper eyelid and is typically not visible unless the upper eyelid is pulled up. Some surgeons may place a small shunt, called an Express shunt, underneath the scleral flap to control the flow of eye fluid—this method is an accepted and effective alternative way of performing trabeculectomy surgery.

GLAUCOMA DRAINAGE DEVICE (TUBE SHUNT) Glaucoma tube shunt surgery may be needed to lower the eye pressure if medications or laser are inadequate or in certain types of glaucoma where conventional surgery would almost certainly fail. It should not be confused with the Express shunt (described above), which is much smaller and placed under the flap of a trabeculectomy. In glaucoma tube surgery, an implant is placed over the sclera but under the conjunctiva, usually in one of the corners of your eye between the eye muscles. The tube connected to this implant is then inserted through the sclera into the eye, allowing fluid to exit. The fluid collects in a pocket formed by the implant and is reabsorbed into nearby blood vessels. The implant and fluid pocket cannot be felt and usually are not visible unless the eyelids are opened widely.

What You May Experience during the Procedure • The procedure is performed in the operating room with the help of a team of nurses and anesthesiologists. Prior to the start of surgery, you will be positioned on your back on the operating bed. The anesthesia team will then attach monitoring devices to watch your heart rate, blood pressure, and oxygen levels throughout the surgery. They will then administer relaxing medication through your veins to keep you comfortably sedated throughout the surgery, but typically you will remain awake. (During the surgery, you may hear the surgeon speak to the assistants.) The area around your eye will be cleaned in a sterile fashion and then plastic surgical drapes will be placed over your whole body, leaving only the operative eye exposed to the surgeon. A speculum will be used to keep your eyelids open during the surgery, so you do not need to worry about blinking during the operation. It is okay to blink the other eye. The eye itself will also be numbed. You may feel some pressure sensations throughout the operation, but should not feel any pain. You should notify your surgeon if you do feel pain. You will not be able to see the surgery. At the end of the surgery, the drapes will be removed and a patch will be placed on the operative eye. You will then be returned to the recovery room prior to being discharged.

Possible Complications • Immediately following most glaucoma surgeries, less so following MIGS, the eye may be sore and the eyelids may be swollen. Over-the-counter pain pills, such as acetaminophen, are usually sufficient to keep you comfortable, but you may feel a foreign body sensation like sand or grit in your eye for the first few days after surgery. The eye may be sore, especially when you look around, due to some bruising. You will also be prescribed eye drops to help the eye heal.

As with any operation, there are risks of bleeding, infection, drooping of the eyelid, retinal detachment, and a possibility that you may need additional operations. Eye pressure after surgery may be too low or too high, leading to a set of complications that can have an impact on vision and recovery. Some eye pressure–related complications may be painless, while others may be associated with a dull aching or throbbing sensation. Your surgeon may change your eye drop regimen or perform special procedures in the clinic to help return your eye pressure to a safe level. In some instances, further surgery in the operating room may be required.

These risks are most likely to occur early on, usually within the first few weeks following the surgery. Over time, excessive scarring during the healing process may result in failure of the operation and increased eye pressure. When this occurs, your eye doctor may adjust your medications, perform procedures in the clinic, or recommend a new surgery to help restore your eye pressure to a safe level. If you have worsening eye pain, eye redness, eye drainage, or decreasing vision, you should notify your eye surgeon as these could be signs of infection, which may occur soon after or even years after surgery. It is important to follow up regularly after any eye surgery to ensure a proper recovery.

Prognosis: Will I See Better? • The goal of glaucoma surgery is to lower your eye pressure in an effort to prevent further vision loss. Vision that has been lost due to glaucoma cannot be restored. Vision may be blurred temporarily after surgery until the eye is healed.

Additional Resources

https://eyewiki.aao.org/Trabeculectomy
https://eyewiki.aao.org/Glaucoma_Drainage_Devices

Minimally Invasive Glaucoma Surgery (MIGS)

SUSAN M. WAKIL, MD

What Is It? • Minimally invasive glaucoma surgery (MIGS) is an umbrella term that includes a variety of procedures that lower eye pressure. These procedures are generally associated with fewer surgical risks than the traditional glaucoma surgeries but also have a more modest reduction in eye pressure. There exist various types of MIGS targeting different pathways to lower eye pressure. You may be a good candidate for one of the MIGS procedures but not necessarily all of them. Eye pressure–reduction outcomes may vary from one patient to another. There are no established guidelines regarding patient selection for each of these procedures. Your surgeon will discuss with you the pros and cons of these procedures, some of which involve implanting special devices to lower eye pressure, and select one that is most appropriate for you based on your glaucoma disease stage and prior ocular history.

ISTENT (GLAUKOS CORP, LAGUNA HILLS, CA) This device is made of titanium and consists of the smallest approved implantable device, approximately 1mm in size, which is inserted into the drainage (trabecular) meshwork of the eye. This device improves outflow of the eye fluid from inside the eye. To date, this device is only approved for use in combination with cataract surgery.

HYDRUS MICROSTENT (IVANTIS INC, IRVINE, CA) This device consists of a small flexible scaffold, approximately the size of an eyelash, made of titanium and nickel. It is implanted circumferentially into the drainage meshwork. This device, like the Istent, reduces your intraocular pressure by improving outflow, but targets a larger surface area.

Of note, neither of these devices will set off airport alarms and both are safe in MRI scanners.

Unlike the above procedures that are meant to enhance aqueous humor drainage, the following procedures are meant to create a new pathway for aqueous humor outflow similar to the traditional trabeculectomy but a less invasive approach.

XEN GEL STENT (ALLERGAN, CA) This device consists of a gel microstent tube. Like trabeculectomy surgery, its purpose is to create a bleb under your conjunctiva, but because it involves an intraocular approach, it is a less-invasive procedure.

INNFOCUS MICROSHUNT/PRESERFLO (SANTEN, OSAKA, JAPAN) This device consists of an arrow-shaped, 8-mm-long tube, made of a biocompatible material called SIBS (Styrene-block-IsoButylene-block-Styrene). It is inserted under your conjunctiva on the upper part of the eye. Like the Xen Gel Stent and traditional trabeculectomy, this device drains fluid from inside the eye to the outside and creates a bleb under your eyelid. This shunt is not yet available for use and is pending FDA approval.

Unlike the other MIGS procedures described above, which involve insertion of a certain device, the following devices do not remain in the eye but instead are used to enlarge the eye's natural drainage pathway in order to improve outflow of the aqueous humor fluid.

TRABECTOME (NEOMEDIX CORP, TUSTIN, CA) The trabectome removes the trabecular meshwork using an electrical pulse and increases the drainage capacity of the eye.

KAHOOK DUAL BLADE (KDB, NEW WORLD MEDICAL, RANCHO CUCAMONGA, CA) The KDB also removes a small segment of the drainage (trabecular) meshwork with the use of a blade that is safe for use inside the eye.

GONIOTOMY-ASSISTED TRANSLUMINAL TRABECULOTOMY (GATT)/ OMNI These procedures involve removal of the diseased drainage (trabecular) meshwork around the whole circumference of the inside of the eye. During the GATT procedure, an illuminated catheter or a thick suture is threaded 360 degrees around the circumference of the eye and is then slowly pulled out from the eye while simultaneously cleaving the trabecular meshwork. OMNI has a similar endpoint but involves a different surgical approach during which the canal is also dilated. Both of these procedures may be associated with more bleeding than the trabectome and KDB.

Unlike all of the above procedures, which aim to increase aqueous fluid outflow in various manners, the following procedure aims to decrease aqueous humor production by directly targeting the ciliary body, the ocular structure responsible for making the aqueous fluid.

ENDOCYCLOPHOTOCOAGULATION (ECP) This procedure consists of a laser probe which is directly aimed at the ciliary body. It is performed in the operating room and requires a small incision to be made in the eye to directly visualize and alter the ciliary body.

Optic Neuritis

JAMES H. POWERS, MD

What Is It? • Optic neuritis is a condition in which the optic nerve, which sends visual information from your eye to your brain, becomes inflamed. This inflammation may lead to vision loss and pain, especially with eye movements. Optic neuritis most commonly occurs in young adult females and may be associated with autoimmune diseases or certain infections; however, it is often idiopathic (i.e., without a specific cause).

Optic neuritis is commonly associated with multiple sclerosis (MS), a condition in which various parts of the central nervous system including the optic nerve become inflamed. It is often the first sign of MS and as many as 50% of MS patients may experience optic neuritis at some point. It may also be associated with a condition known as neuromyelitis optica (NMO), another condition involving inflammation of the optic nerve and spinal cord.

Symptoms: What You May Experience • Optic neuritis often results in diminished vision, which may include general blurring of vision, difficulty distinguishing colors, or dark areas in the field of vision. Eye pain, especially with eye movement, is also common in optic neuritis.

Examination Findings: What the Doctor Looks For • Your eye doctor will perform a complete eye exam, including a dilated eye exam to evaluate the optic nerve and retina in the back of your eye. Your eye doctor will perform tests to evaluate your visual acuity, color vision, and side (or peripheral) vision. They will also examine your pupils and eye movements. Because optic neuritis may signal a more widespread inflammatory condition occurring in the body, your doctor may also order blood tests, a magnetic resonance imaging (MRI) scan of your brain and orbits, or sometimes even a lumbar puncture ("spinal tap") to check for inflammation in the fluid that surrounds your brain and spinal cord.

What You Can Do • There is currently no proven way to prevent optic neuritis. If you believe you are experiencing optic neuritis, contact your eye doctor and also inform them of any other symptoms you may be experiencing that could indicate a more widespread inflammatory condition.

When to Call the Doctor • If you are experiencing eye pain, decreased vision, or difficulty distinguishing colors, contact your eye doctor promptly for an evaluation. If you have already been diagnosed with optic neuritis and your symptoms change, worsen, persist, or recur, you should also contact your eye doctor. Prompt medical attention is the best way to ensure optimal outcomes.

Treatment • Often, optic neuritis resolves on its own after several weeks and does not need treatment. Occasionally, your eye doctor may recommend steroid medications which are given intravenously (by vein) that may result in earlier restoration of vision. However, the long-term visual outcome is the same with or without steroids. In rare cases of optic neuritis that persist despite the passage of time and steroid treatment, a treatment called plasma exchange therapy may be attempted to recover some vision.

Prognosis: Will I See Better? • Most patients with optic neuritis recover vision, either partially or fully. Rarely, some may experience permanent vision loss. In those with a history of optic neuritis, there is a chance that optic neuritis may recur in the same eye or the fellow eye.

Additional Resources

https://eyewiki.aao.org/Demyelinating_Optic_Neuritis

https://www.aao.org/eye-health/diseases/optic-neuritis-diagnosis

Papilledema

JAMES H. POWERS, MD

What Is It? • Papilledema is a condition in which the optic nerve, which is the structure that connects the eye to the brain, becomes swollen due to elevated intracranial pressure. The fluid that surrounds the brain, called the cerebrospinal fluid (CSF), also surrounds the optic nerve, thus increases in CSF pressure may also affect the optic nerve.

Papilledema may be caused by any factor that increases the intracranial pressure, including a tumor or bleed inside the skull, brain swelling, trauma, too much CSF, blood-flow problems, medication side effects, and idiopathic intracranial hypertension (IIH). IIH is a condition with signs and symptoms of elevated intracranial pressure without any known cause.

Symptoms: What You May Experience • You may experience brief episodes of visual blackout or dimming. These episodes may affect one or both eyes, may involve all or part of the visual field, and may last only a few seconds at a time. Other symptoms may include double vision, headaches (especially worse lying down and waking up in the morning), nausea, vomiting, and pulsatile machine-like "whooshing" sound in one or both ears. Sometimes, papilledema is discovered on an eye exam before symptoms arise. It is important to report any of the above symptoms to your eye doctor, as untreated papilledema may lead to permanent vision loss.

Examination Findings: What the Doctor Looks For • Your eye doctor will perform a complete eye exam, including a dilated eye exam. Your doctor will check your visual acuity, color vision, side (peripheral) vision, eye movements, and pupils. After dilating your pupils with eye drops, your doctor will examine your optic nerve and retina in the back part of the eye, particularly checking for any swelling of the optic nerve. If the optic nerves in both eyes are swollen, your eye doctor will order magnetic resonance imaging (MRI) of your brain and orbits to determine possible causes for papilledema. Your doctor may also order a lumbar puncture (also known as a spinal tap) to measure the CSF pressure and obtain a sample of CSF for analysis. In certain cases, your eye doctor may order blood tests to investigate other possible causes of papilledema.

In the clinic, your eye doctor may order eye-imaging tests such as optical coherence tomography (OCT) and color photographs to help monitor and analyze the swelling of your optic nerves in response to treatment.

What You Can Do • Some causes of papilledema and elevated intracranial pressure are difficult to prevent. Idiopathic intracranial hypertension is often associated with obesity, therefore maintaining a healthy weight through diet and exercise may prevent this cause of elevated intracranial pressure. Any trauma to the head accompanied by vision loss should prompt you to seek medical attention, as bleeding inside the skull may elevate intracranial pressure.

When to Call the Doctor • If you experience decreased vision, episodes of vision loss/darkening, double vision, headaches that are worse in the morning or when lying down, you should contact your eye doctor promptly.

Treatment • The treatment for papilledema and elevated intracranial pressure depends on the underlying cause. If papilledema is the result of idiopathic intracranial hypertension, treatment will likely involve use of the medication acetazolamide (Diamox) as well as weight loss. In more severe cases, surgery may be required to prevent permanent vision loss. Surgeries may include opening the sheath surrounding the optic nerve, or placing a shunt to help drain CSF and lower intracranial pressure. If the elevated intracranial pressure is due to a medication side effect, your eye doctor will likely discontinue the medication. If a tumor is the cause, medical and/or surgical treatment of the tumor may be required. In all cases, treatment for papilledema should be initiated promptly.

Prognosis: Will I See Better? • Papilledema is often successfully treated with prompt medical attention. However, permanent vision loss due to optic nerve damage may occur if papilledema is not treated early enough. Factors that are associated with a worse visual prognosis include older age, high blood pressure, anemia (low blood counts), and glaucoma. It is essential to diagnose and treat papilledema as soon as possible.

Additional Resource

https://eyewiki.aao.org/Papilledema

Strabismus (Misaligned Eyes)

LAURA B. ENYEDI, MD

What Is It? • Strabismus is a condition in which the eyes are not pointed in the same direction. One or both eyes may cross in toward the nose (esotropia), out toward the ear (exotropia), upward (hypertropia), or downward (hypotropia). The misalignment may be constant or may come and go, varying from day to day or even over the course of a day. The misalignment may be the same no matter where the eyes are looking or may be better or worse in different directions of gaze or when looking far away or close up.

Strabismus can occur at any age and is common, affecting 2–5% of the population. Strabismus is often seen in children and may be present in infancy or develop in the first few years of life. The cause of most childhood strabismus is unknown.

Eye movements are normally controlled by six muscles that are attached to each eye. The brain coordinates the actions of all twelve muscles so that they work together to point both eyes in the same direction. Children with disorders that affect the brain such as cerebral palsy, Down syndrome, hydrocephalus, or brain tumors are more likely to develop strabismus than other children. There is also an increased risk of strabismus in children who have a family history of strabismus, who are born prematurely, or who have other eye disorders such as cataract.

Symptoms: What You May Experience • Normal alignment of the eyes is critical for normal visual development. Strabismus in children is often associated with poor visual development (amblyopia) in one eye, which may be permanent. Strabismus also interferes with the ability to use the eyes together and can affect depth perception. Young children do not usually notice any problems with their vision and will often have no symptoms other than a tendency for one or both eyes to point the wrong direction. Sometimes, a child will squint one eye in bright sunlight or ab-

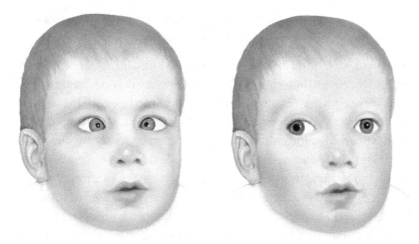

15.1. Left: the eyes cross in toward the nose in esotropia. Right: the eyes drift out toward the ears in exotropia.

normally turn or tilt their head because of the strabismus. In older children and adults, strabismus may cause double vision (diplopia).

Examination Findings: What the Doctor Looks For • Anyone with strabismus needs a full eye exam, including infants who can be examined using specialized techniques. The eye doctor will determine how the eyes are working together, the amount of the misalignment, the vision in each eye, and the refraction (glasses prescription). The eyes will be dilated and fully examined for other serious diseases such as cataracts or eye tumors that can cause strabismus in children.

What You Can Do • Strabismus is not a preventable condition.

When to Call the Doctor • It is critical that childhood strabismus be diagnosed and treated early. If you suspect that your child has strabismus, you should immediately take them to an eye doctor (preferably a pediatric eye specialist) for a full examination. The eyes of a very young infant often do not focus together and may occasionally wander, but after the age of 3 months, your child's eyes should focus together and be aligned. If the eyes are not straight by this age, your child should undergo an eye exam. An adult who develops strabismus or double vision also needs a prompt examination by an eye doctor to diagnose possible serious diseases such as brain tumor or stroke that can cause eye misalignments.

Treatment • Strabismus is not outgrown and usually does not improve without treatment. In young children, early treatment is critical for proper vision development. Various treatments may be used alone or in combination, depending on the type and cause of the strabismus. Strabismus treatment is often combined with amblyopia treatment. Glasses are sometimes helpful for childhood strabismus. In adults, double vision can sometimes be relieved by using prisms in the glasses. Occasionally, medications in the form of eye drops or injections into the eye muscles are used to treat strabismus. Surgery to realign the eye muscles is frequently necessary for both children and adults. Often, both eyes require eye muscle surgery, and more than one surgery may be necessary to align the eyes.

Prognosis: Will I See Better? • With proper prompt treatment, strabismus can be corrected or alleviated in many cases. In children, treatment of strabismus can prevent the development of amblyopia.

Additional Resources

www.aapos.org

www.preventblindness.org

Amblyopia (Lazy Eye)

NATHAN CHEUNG, OD, FAAO

What Is It? • Amblyopia, or "lazy eye," is decreased eyesight in one or both eyes due to abnormal visual development. Amblyopia develops during the first 7–9 years of life. As children begin to use their eyes, the region of the brain responsible for vision also begins to develop. If there is something that prevents the child's vision from developing properly, then amblyopia occurs.

There are three main causes/categories of amblyopia. The first category is refractive amblyopia, where one or both eyes needs a very strong glasses prescription (the prescription can be for nearsightedness, farsightedness, or astigmatism) but the child doesn't wear one. Due to the need for a strong prescription, the child is not able to see well, and the region of the brain responsible for vision does not develop properly.

The second category is strabismic amblyopia. Strabismic amblyopia occurs when the eyes are misaligned (strabismus). Due to the strabismus, the child subconsciously "turns off" or suppresses the wandering/misaligned eye, thus the visual pathway does not develop in the suppressed eye.

The third category is deprivation amblyopia. Deprivation amblyopia occurs when there is something that blocks the vision to an eye. This can be caused by a droopy eyelid, a cloudy cornea, or a cataract. Due to a lack of visual input in the affected eye, the visual pathway does not develop properly in that eye.

Symptoms: What You May Experience • Adults with amblyopia either have one eye that sees worse than the other or poor vision in both eyes. This poor vision cannot be corrected by glasses, medication, or surgery since the problem is related to poor visual brain development.

Children with amblyopia may or may not notice poor vision in one eye. Parentos may notice crossing or drifting eyes, or whiteness of the pupil. However, most young children do not voice any complaints about their eyes; therefore, it is important to have regular eye exams.

Examination Findings: What the Doctor Looks for • The eye doctor will evaluate the eye by checking visual acuity, looking for any eye misalignment, and making sure that the eyes are healthy. A complete eye exam with pupil dilation is essential to rule out other causes of decreased vision.

When to Call the Doctor • If you are the parent of a young child, you should have your child examined by an eye doctor if you notice that they have crossing or drifting eyes, a white-looking pupil, difficulty performing vision tasks, or any other eye abnormality.

Treatment • If diagnosed early enough, the treatment for amblyopia consists of forcing the child to use the "lazy" eye. Usually, this is accomplished by patching the preferred or good eye for several hours a day. Additionally, atropine eye drops and special glasses can be used to blur the good eye and thus encourage the child to use the amblyopic eye. If a cataract is present, surgical removal of the cataract may be required before amblyopia can improve. Eye muscle surgery to correct eye misalignment may be done before or after patching therapy. In all cases, frequent followup visits with the eye doctor are necessary to monitor changes in vision.

Will I (or Will My Child) See Better? • Success in treating amblyopia depends on two factors: the severity of visual loss and the age at which therapy is started. The earlier amblyopia is diagnosed and treated, the more likely vision will improve. Once vision has improved, maintenance therapy may be necessary until the child is past the amblyogenic age (7 to 9 years old). Adult patients cannot improve amblyopic vision.

Additional Resources

http://www.preventblindness.org/children/amblyopiaFAQ.html
http://www.nei.nih.gov/health/amblyopia
http://www.aapos.org/

Orbital Cellulitis

HENRY L. FENG, MD

What Is It? • Orbital cellulitis is an infection in the orbit, or eye socket, that can cause vision loss as well as serious complications elsewhere in the body. Swelling due to infection in the orbit may cause increased pressure on the eyeball, blood vessels, and optic nerve, leading to vision loss. Orbital cellulitis is usually caused by a bacterial infection that spreads either from the sinuses or from an eyelid infection into the orbit. Sinus disease is the most common cause of orbital cellulitis because multiple sinuses are located next to the orbit, separated only by thin bone. Serious sinus infections can spread into the orbit through these thin bones. In some cases of orbital cellulitis, an abscess, or pus collection, may form.

Another cause of orbital cellulitis is the spread of infection from the eyelids and surrounding skin, which is called preseptal cellulitis. Although preseptal cellulitis can be severe, it is usually not vision-threatening. However, if not treated promptly, this infection can sometimes penetrate the orbital septum, a thin layer of tissue behind the eyelids that normally helps prevent skin infections from reaching the orbit. Once the infection crosses this natural barrier, orbital cellulitis can result.

Symptoms: What You May Experience • Swelling of the eyelid, eye redness, eye discharge, and eye pain are early signs of preseptal or orbital cellulitis. A fever may or may not be present. Double vision, difficulty or significant pain with eye movements, decreased vision, or an eye that bulges forward often signifies severe orbital involvement.

Examination Findings: What the Doctor Looks For • Your eye doctor will perform a comprehensive eye exam, including pupillary dilation, to look for signs of infection in the eyelids, surrounding skin, and orbit. A sample of pus-like discharge may be collected to determine what type of bacteria may be causing the infection. When orbital cellulitis is suspected, blood tests and neuroimaging (typically a CT scan) of the brain and orbits are often performed.

What You Can Do • If you have sinus disease or an eyelid infection, see your doctor to make sure these conditions are properly treated so that they do not spread and result in orbital cellulitis.

When to Call the Doctor • If you notice eyelid swelling, eye redness, or eye pain, you should contact your eye doctor for an evaluation. If you have decreased vision, pus-like discharge from the eye, double vision, difficulty with eye movements, or an eye that bulges forward, you should be examined promptly by your eye doctor or the nearest emergency department.

Treatment • Orbital cellulitis is usually treated with intravenous antibiotics in the hospital. If an abscess has formed or the orbital cellulitis is not responding to antibiotics, surgery may be required to drain the infection. Preseptal cellulitis is usually treated with oral antibiotics, and hospitalization may or may not be necessary depending on the severity of the infection. Frequent monitoring of both of these conditions is important during recovery.

Prognosis: Will I See Better? • The prognosis of orbital cellulitis depends on the extent and severity of the infection. In many cases, your vision will likely return to normal after the infection resolves with proper treatment. If uncontrolled, however, the infection may spread beyond the orbit and reach the brain. Death is an extremely rare complication of severe, untreated orbital cellulitis.

Additional Resource

https://eyewiki.aao.org/Orbital_Cellulitis

Thyroid Eye Disease

ROSHNI RANJIT-REEVES, MD

What Is It? • The thyroid gland is a butterfly-shaped gland located at the front of the neck; it is a vital organ that controls the body's metabolism, growth, and development through the production of thyroid hormone. Thyroid dysfunction is often identified using lab tests that measure the amount of thyroid hormone in the blood. Thyroid eye disease, sometimes referred to as Graves' disease, is an autoimmune inflammatory condition that can occur if you have a thyroid gland that is overactive (hyperthyroid), underactive (hypothyroid), or normal (euthyroid). It can also be associated with another autoimmune condition called myasthenia gravis, which can cause muscle weakness. Thyroid eye disease occurs in 16 out of 100,000 people per year for women and 2.9 out of 100,000 people per year for men. It occurs most commonly in the 5th and 7th decades of life, and about 3–5% of cases are vision-threatening.

Symptoms: What You May Experience • Your eyes may appear to be enlarged or bulging forward. You may have difficulty moving your eyes in certain directions and may also experience double vision (diplopia), eye dryness, eye swelling, and decreased vision.

Examination Findings: What the Doctor Looks For • Your eye doctor will perform a comprehensive eye exam, including a dilated eye exam, and will measure the degree of bulging (proptosis) with a special eye ruler and evaluate your vision, pupils, eye movements, eye pressure, and color vision. Your doctor will check for eye dryness, and after dilation, examine the retina and optic nerves for any evidence of damage. If your eye doctor suspects thyroid eye disease, neuroimaging will be ordered, typically a CT scan or MRI scan of the brain and orbits, to look at your eye muscles and optic nerve within the orbit. Additional blood tests may also be collected to check levels of thyroid stimulating antibodies in the blood.

What You Can Do • Regular followup with your primary care doctor to evaluate and manage any thyroid dysfunction is important. Smoking may lead to worsening of thyroid eye disease; therefore, you should avoid or stop smoking.

When to Call the Doctor • It is important to tell your primary care physician if you notice any changes in your health or evidence of changes in your metabolism such as unexplained weight gain or loss. Contact your eye doctor if you notice vision changes, eye irritation, eye redness, double vision, bulging eyes, or difficulty distinguishing colors. Prompt treatment can decrease the chance of permanent damage caused by severe thyroid eye disease.

Treatment • Treatment options vary depending on the severity of the disease. Lubricating eye drops or eye ointment may help treat and prevent dry eye symptoms. Oral steroids can be given to lessen inflammation of tissues within the orbit. Chemotherapy agents, radiation, and/or intravenous high dose steroids are usually reserved for more advanced disease. If you have double vision due to thyroid eye disease, prism glasses can be used as a temporary measure to improve double vision until the disease has been treated and stabilized. Surgical treatment may be considered for cases in which the disease has stabilized to allow for more predictable results. Surgical options include orbital decompression to provide more space for the swollen tissues, eye muscle surgery for double vision or eye misalignment, and eyelid surgery to improve the position of the upper and lower eyelids. It is important to work closely with your eye doctor, endocrine specialist, and primary care doctor as this disease can affect multiple organs in the body.

Prognosis: Will I See Better? • The prognosis depends largely on the severity and duration of the disease. While permanent vision loss can occur from optic nerve compression, it is rare. It is important to work closely with your eye doctor so that vision, functionality, and cosmetic appearance can be addressed. Thyroid eye disease can affect your quality of life, but management can improve ocular health and save vision if addressed early.

Additional Resource

https://eyewiki.aao.org/Thyroid_Ophthalmopathy

Orbital Ecchymosis (Black Eye)

HERB GREENMAN, MD

What Is It? • Orbital ecchymosis, or black eye, is a collection of fluid and blood in the tissues around the eye (orbit), leading to swelling and discoloration of the overlying eyelid skin. Orbital ecchymosis can be thought of as bruising around the eye and is usually caused by trauma or surgery to the eyes, nose, or face. Bilateral deep orbital ecchymosis (raccoon eyes) from head trauma can be a sign of a basilar skull fracture. Rarely, orbital ecchymosis can be caused by tumors, amyloidosis, bleeding disorders, or blood-thinning medications.

Symptoms: What You May Experience • You may experience swelling and reddish discoloration of the eyelids and tissues surrounding the eye. The swelling and discoloration may expand before resolving, and the area may ultimately turn purple, yellow, green, or black. The vision may or may not be affected.

Examination Findings: What the Doctor Looks For • The eye doctor will ask about any trauma to the eye and then look for any associated injuries such as a penetrating eye wound or orbital wall fracture. The doctor will perform a full eye exam including a dilated eye exam to look for injuries in and around the eye. Special x-rays or a CT scan may be performed to look for bone fractures or foreign bodies.

What You Can Do • If the bruising is due to a blunt eye injury, you can apply ice to your closed eyelids for 20 minutes every hour while awake for the first 24–48 hours after an injury to reduce the amount of swelling. Do not apply ice or pressure to the eye if you think an object has penetrated or perforated your eyeball.

When to Call the Doctor • Bruising around the eye typically resolves spontaneously; however, you should seek medical attention immediately if you think something has pierced the eye or if there are large cuts to the eye area. Concerning symptoms that should prompt you to visit the emergency department include decreased or double vision, loss of consciousness, blood or clear fluid from the nose or ears, blood on the surface of the eye, persistent headache, severe pain, and any symptom that is worsening. You should also see an eye doctor soon after bruising occurs if the swelling does not improve over several days, if the area of injury appears infected, or if the ecchymosis is not the result of an injury. In orbital ecchymosis due to an eye injury, you should follow up with an eye doctor even after the bruising has resolved, because you may be at risk for glaucoma or other eye problems.

Treatment • Treatment depends on the type of injuries incurred with a black eye. The black eye itself is normally treated with ice packs for the first 24–48 hours after the injury.

Prognosis: Will I See Better? • Over 1–2 weeks, the bruising of the skin will become lighter and the swelling will subside. Bruising around the eye does not usually affect vision; however, the visual outcome varies depending on the extent of any associated eye injuries.

Additional Resource

https://www.aao.org/eye-health/diseases/black-eye

Hyphema

HERB GREENMAN, MD

What Is It? • A hyphema is blood in the anterior chamber of the front of the eye, between the iris and cornea. It may be the result of an eye injury or eye surgery, or could occur spontaneously. Spontaneous causes may include abnormal blood vessels growing on the iris, tumors in the eye, or bleeding disorders. Abnormal blood vessels on the iris may be triggered by lack of blood supply to the eye, diabetes, inflammation, or retinal detachment. Hyphema may cause elevated eye pressure and could cause blood staining of the cornea, if untreated.

Symptoms: What You May Experience • Common symptoms of hyphema include blurred vision and eye pain. Layering blood may be visible inside the anterior chamber of the eye.

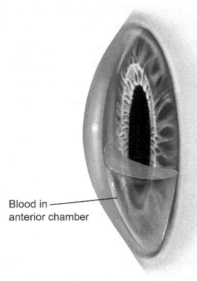

Blood in
anterior chamber

17.1. Blood fills the anterior chamber in a hyphema.

Examination Findings: What the Doctor Looks For • The eye doctor will inquire about any recent eye injury or eye surgery. They will perform a complete eye exam which will include checking your eye pressure and looking for blood in the anterior chamber using a slit lamp microscope. African Americans, Hispanics, and those of Mediterranean descent should be screened for sickle cell trait or disease, since patients with sickle cell are more likely to have permanent eye damage from a hyphema.

What You Can Do • Avoid eye injury to lessen your risk of developing a hyphema. Wear appropriate eye protection when performing high-risk activities such as contact sports or work involving projectiles or machinery.

When to Call the Doctor • If you notice blurred vision or eye pain following trauma or recent eye surgery, contact your eye doctor as soon as possible.

Treatment • Cycloplegic (dilating) and steroid eye drops may be given to lessen inflammation in the eye, and pressure-lowering eye drops may be needed to control the eye pressure. Pain can be managed with oral acetaminophen; aspirin and other nonsteroidal anti-inflammatory drugs (NSAIDs) such as ibuprofen should be avoided unless absolutely necessary as these drugs can contribute to re-bleeding. If you are at an increased risk for re-bleeding, you may be placed on topical or oral aminocaproic acid (Amicar). You may be instructed to sleep with your head elevated and refrain from strenuous activity so that the blood can settle to the bottom of the anterior chamber. Rarely, hospitalization may be needed for close monitoring of vision and eye pressure, especially in children.

Usually a hyphema will be naturally reabsorbed by your body. However, surgery to remove the blood clot may be indicated if the hyphema is large and lasts for more than 5–10 days, if the cornea is at risk for being stained by blood, or if the eye pressure cannot be controlled with medications.

Prognosis: Will I See Better? • In many cases, the vision will improve as the hyphema resolves. If the eye pressure was extremely high for a very long time when the hyphema occurred, the optic nerve could be damaged, which may permanently affect your vision. In cases of blunt eye injury, visual potential usually depends on the extent of the initial injury.

Additional Resource

https://eyewiki.aao.org/Hyphema

Orbital Fracture

KENNETH NEUFELD, MD, ANNA GINTER, MD,
AND JULIE A. WOODWARD, MD

What Is It? • An orbital fracture (sometimes called a "blow-out" fracture) is a broken bone in any of the bony walls of the orbit, which is the "eye socket" where the eyeball rests. When trauma to the area around the eye occurs, forces are transmitted through the orbit and may cause the bones to break and literally "blow out" into the surrounding sinuses. Of the four bony walls of the orbit, the medial wall (next to the nose) and the bottom wall (known as the orbital floor) are the weakest and most commonly broken during orbital trauma.

Symptoms: What You May Experience • If you have had a blunt injury to your eye or the area around your eye and have been diagnosed with an orbital fracture, you may have pain in your face or eye, swelling, bruising, and possibly a nosebleed. The affected eye may have restricted movement and you may experience double vision when trying to look up, down, left, or right. There may be numbness of the cheek, upper lip, or teeth on the affected side. These symptoms occur because a muscle or nerve may have been injured as a result of the fracture. The affected eye may also appear to have a sunken position compared to the unaffected eye.

Examination Findings: What the Doctor Looks For • Besides checking for injuries in other parts of your body, your doctor will check your vision and eye movements. Your eyes will also be examined to see if the eyeball itself has been injured. If an orbital fracture is suspected, your doctor may order imaging such as a computed tomography (CT) scan to confirm the diagnosis.

What You Can Do • The best way to avoid an orbital fracture is to avoid blunt trauma to the eye and face. Use appropriate protective eyewear in situations where eye injury is possible.

When to Call the Doctor • If you have been hit in the eye or area around your eye, you should seek prompt medical attention at your closest emergency room.

Treatment • In most orbital fracture cases, ice packs should be applied to the face and eye as often as tolerated for the first 48 hours. You should also avoid blowing your nose and may be prescribed a nasal decongestant spray and oral antibiotics to help decrease the chance of infection.

Surgical repair of an orbital fracture often does not need to be per formed immediately, since swelling, bleeding, and double vision may resolve spontaneously after 1 to 4 weeks. Some small fractures do not need surgery at all. In many cases, treatment may be done on an out-patient basis, with hospital admission needed in just over half of cases. Signs that may warrant earlier surgery include double vision when looking straight ahead or downward, a sunken position of the affected eyeball that is 2 mm or greater compared to the other eye, or a slowed heart rate caused by the eye injury, which can (rarely) occur if an eye muscle becomes trapped. In repairing the fracture, the surgeon will attempt to remove any tissues trapped within the fractured bones and will place a new orbital wall, which may be made out of bone or synthetic material, to support the broken area. You should see your eye doctor periodically after this type of injury to make sure that the fracture heals properly and that no late complications develop, such as double vision or glaucoma.

Prognosis: Will I See Better? • The prognosis for vision and facial appearance depends on the extent of the initial injury. Many patients recover well after treatment.

Additional Resources

https://eyewiki.aao.org/Orbital_Floor_Fractures

https://www.asoprs.org/orbital—blow-out—fractures

Open Globe

CASSANDRA C. BROOKS, MD

What Is It? • An open or ruptured globe is when the eye has a full thickness cut or wound and is no longer a fully intact globe or compartment. This may be very subtle or very apparent depending on the extent of the injury. Many mechanisms can lead to an open globe, including motor vehicle accidents, fights, sporting injuries, or any hard object making forceful contact with the eye. Objects may cause penetrating injuries (entry wound only) and then remain within the eye, resulting in an intraocular foreign body, or they may cause perforating injuries (entry and exit wounds). Other eye injuries can occur with an open globe, including broken facial bones, cataract, bleeding, and retinal detachment.

Symptoms: What You May Experience • Often, severe open globe injuries result in severely decreased vision and eye pain. The eye may appear deformed and may also have associated bleeding or leaking of intraocular contents.

Examination Findings: What the Doctor Looks For • Your eye doctor will perform a careful eye examination if an open globe is suspected. They will check your vision and examine your eye using a slit lamp microscope to see if a full thickness cut or opening is present. Sometimes, the eye pressure and eye movements will not be assessed as these exam maneuvers could cause more intraocular contents to extrude. Usually, a computed tomography (CT) scan or other imaging modality of the eyes and orbits is performed to help determine if there is an intraocular foreign body.

What You Can Do • Eye protection is the key to minimizing your risk of an open globe injury. During high-risk activities, such as sports or lawn mowing, it is important to wear safety glasses to protect yourself from an eye injury from projectiles or forceful contact with hard objects.

When to Call the Doctor • If you suspect an open globe injury has occurred, you should seek immediate evaluation at the nearest emergency department. Do not eat or drink anything in case surgery is required. If possible, without placing excess pressure or touching the eye, tape a plastic or Styrofoam cup over the eye with the open end toward the eye. This can help protect the eye from further injury. Try your best to avoid blowing your nose, coughing, sneezing, or bearing down because these activities can increase the pressure in your head and could extrude contents from an eye that is open.

Treatment • Emergency surgery within 24 hours is usually performed to repair an open globe and remove any intraocular foreign bodies. The goal of closing the eye is to prevent further injury and decrease the risk of eye infection. Even with successful closure of the eye, additional surgeries may be required in the future to treat traumatic cataracts, bleeding within the eye, or a retinal detachment. After surgery, eye drops and oral medications may be prescribed to help decrease pain, inflammation, and the chance of infection.

Prognosis: Will I See Better? • Eye surgeons are usually able to successfully close a ruptured globe; however, visual outcomes vary widely based on the extent of the injury. If the eye injury is severe enough, it might not be possible to repair the eye and it may need to be removed instead. In these cases, an implant will be placed in the eye socket and a non-seeing prosthesis can be made to match the other eye.

Additional Resources

https://eyewiki.aao.org/Ocular_penetrating_and_perforating_injuries
https://eyewiki.aao.org/Intraocular_Foreign_Bodies_(IOFB)

Foreign Body

CASSANDRA C. BROOKS, MD

What Is It? • A foreign body is an object that is not normally on or in the eye. Foreign bodies can be on the surface of the eye or inside the eye (intraocular foreign body). Things such as metal, wood, glass, or contact lenses can be foreign bodies. Intraocular foreign bodies can be associated with many other eye conditions, including corneal abrasions and open globes.

Symptoms: What You May Experience • Foreign bodies can cause discomfort ranging from a "scratchy or gritty" sensation to significant eye pain depending on the size and location of the object. You could also have eye redness, tearing, light sensitivity, or bleeding.

Examination Findings: What the Doctor Looks For • Your eye doctor will perform a thorough eye exam, including a dilated exam, to determine whether there is a foreign body and whether it is on the surface or inside the eye. A fluorescent eye drop may be used during the exam and your doctor may need to flip the eyelids to check for any objects that might be hidden underneath. A computed tomography (CT) scan or other imaging modality of the eyes and orbits may be obtained if there is concern for an intraocular foreign body that is not readily visible on examination.

What You Can Do • Eye protection is the key to minimizing your risk of acquiring a foreign body. Individuals with high-risk jobs, such as those involving projectiles, heavy machinery, or construction, should wear safety glasses when appropriate. If you suspect a mild surface foreign body such as an eyelash or small piece of sand, you can attempt to remove it by flushing the eye with clean water or artificial tears. Do not rub or apply pressure to the eye as this may cause further injury. Persistent symptoms should warrant a full eye exam.

When to Call the Doctor • If you are unable to flush out a surface foreign body or believe you have an intraocular foreign body, call your eye doctor promptly or go to the emergency room.

Treatment • Surface foreign bodies can often be removed in the emergency department at a slit lamp microscope with the use of an anesthetic eye drop. Surgery is required to remove an intraocular foreign body. Following removal of the foreign body, eye drops or ointment may be recommended to promote healing and decrease the risk of infection.

Prognosis: Will I See Better? • Visual prognosis is variable and largely based on the size, extent, and location of the injury. Small surface foreign bodies may cause temporary visual blurring and tearing but are unlikely to cause permanent vision loss if not associated with an infection or other associated eye injury. Intraocular foreign bodies, particularly associated with a perforating eye injury, can result in visual loss and even loss of the eye.

Additional Resources

https://eyewiki.org/Removal_of_Corneal_Foreign_Bodies

https://eyewiki.aao.org/Intraocular_Foreign_Bodies_(IOFB)

Chemical Injury

JAMES H. POWERS, MD

What Is It? • Chemical injuries can occur when a chemical is splashed onto the eye. These most often occur as accidental exposures in the workplace and may happen even with the use of safety glasses. Alkali burns (e.g., lye, drain cleaners, industrial and household cleaners, fertilizers, cement, plaster) tend to be more severe than acid burns (e.g., hydrochloric acid, battery acid), although both may cause serious eye injury.

Symptoms: What You May Experience • After a chemical splash to the eye, you may experience eye pain, redness, tearing, light sensitivity, and decreased vision.

Examination Findings: What the Doctor Looks For • After exposure to a chemical splash, your eye doctor will flush your eye with salt water (saline) solution until the pH has normalized. They will then perform a comprehensive eye exam to determine the extent and severity of the chemical injury.

What You Can Do • If you are in an environment where you believe there is potential risk of chemical injury to your eyes, be sure to always wear appropriate eye protection. If you believe you may have experienced a chemical injury to the eye, immediately flush the exposed eye with water and ask someone to call 911. *Continue flushing until help arrives.* When you go to the eye doctor, bring a sample of the solution that came into contact with your eye(s).

When to Call the Doctor • Call your eye doctor or 911 immediately after you have experienced a chemical splash to the eye.

Treatment • Primary treatment will involve flushing the chemical out of the eye with saline solution. Any additional treatment will depend on the extent of injury—this may include antibiotic eye drops, lubricating eye drops, and even surgery.

Prognosis: Will I See Better? • Prognosis depends on the extent of injury, the type of chemical, and the length of exposure. Most will experience marked improvement after removal of the offending chemical from the eye and extensive flushing of the eye to normalize the pH level.

Additional Resources

https://www.aao.org/eyenet/article/treating-acute-chemical-injuries-of-cornea

https://eyewiki.aao.org/Chemical_(Alkali_and_Acid)_Injury_of_the_Conjunctiva
   _and_Cornea

Eyelid Lacerations

CASSANDRA C. BROOKS, MD

What Is It? • An eyelid laceration is a cut in or tear of the eyelid. Eyelid lacerations occur from many different mechanisms of injury, including fights, motor vehicle accidents, sporting injuries, or any sharp or blunt object making forceful contact with the eyelid skin. This type of injury can be associated with numerous other eye conditions, including open globes and facial bone fractures.

Symptoms: What You May Experience • Common symptoms include pain, bleeding, and swelling around the site of injury, which may cause decreased vision. Depending on the extent of the injury, the eyelid may appear deformed.

Examination Findings: What the Doctor Looks For • A thorough examination is needed to determine the depth and extent of injury. Your eye doctor will check whether the injury involves the margin of the eyelid and may probe to check the integrity of the nearby tear drainage system. Given the complex structure and function of the eyelid, careful examination is required to develop the best plan for repair. It is also important to determine whether any other eye injuries, such as an open globe or intraocular foreign body, have occurred that would warrant more urgent attention.

What You Can Do • Eye protection is the key to minimizing your risk of an eyelid laceration. Individuals with high-risk jobs, such as those involving projectiles, heavy machinery, or other high-risk activities, should wear appropriate safety glasses. If your eyelid or eyeball becomes injured, avoiding touching it and seek medical attention promptly. If a piece of eyelid is missing, locate it, put it on ice, and bring it to the emergency room.

When to Call the Doctor • If you have injured your eyelid, visit the nearest emergency department for evaluation.

Treatment • It may be possible to clean and repair simple surface lacerations in the emergency department with stitches and local anesthetic. However, more complex eyelid injuries may need to be repaired in the operating room. Injuries involving the eyelid margin require careful correction to prevent malalignment and indentation, which could prevent the eyelids from closing properly, leading to abnormal tearing and corneal irritation. Injuries involving the inner corner of the eyelids may damage the tear drainage system and require careful repair with a silicone tube to prevent the tear drainage canal from scarring closed. The silicone tube is normally removed around 3–6 months after surgery. Following surgery, an antibiotic ointment will be prescribed to decrease the risk of infection and promote healing. Even with the appropriate initial repair, it is possible that future surgeries may be required.

Prognosis: Will I See Better? • Small eyelid lacerations without other injuries do not usually lead to long-term vision problems, and repair often results in a satisfactory cosmetic result. The more complex the eyelid injury, the greater the risk of scarring. Significant scarring can cause the eyelid to be incorrectly positioned, resulting in abnormal tearing or corneal irritation. For injuries involving the tear drainage system, excessive tearing may occur even with proper initial repair, and additional eyelid surgeries may be needed.

Additional Resource

https://eyewiki.aao.org/Eyelid_Laceration

Ocular Prosthesis (Artificial or "Glass" Eye)

KENNETH NEUFELD, MD, ANNA GINTER, MD,

AND JULIE A. WOODWARD, MD

What Is an Ocular Prosthesis? • An ocular prosthesis is a medical term for a non-seeing artificial eye, sometimes referred to as a "glass" eye. Until the 1950s, most ocular prostheses were made out of glass; however, it is now more common for them to be made out of acrylic. Current ocular prostheses are crafted and painted by specialists known as ocularists and look almost identical to normal, healthy eyes. The prosthetic eye does not provide any vision, but instead, it is used to resemble the appearance of a "normal" eye and improve appearance.

The part of the prosthesis that is visible is called a shell. This shell can be placed over a damaged eye, a shrunken eye, or more commonly, an orbital implant. An implant is a sphere made of plastic, silicone, or hydroxyapatite (a material derived from sea coral) which is surgically placed in the orbit at the time that a sick eye is removed and is meant to stay in place permanently. The implant is needed to maintain orbital volume. You will be able to move the prosthetic eye somewhat, but probably not as easily or fully compared to a normal, healthy eye. Motility can sometimes be improved if a connecting peg is placed in the implant and connected to the overlying shell.

Why Are Ocular Protheses Needed? • People may have prosthetic eyes for a variety of reasons. The most common reason to remove a natural, blind eye is to relieve pain. A blind, painful eye may be replaced with a prosthetic eye to relieve symptoms. In other cases, an eye may be damaged beyond repair after severe trauma, and the eye may need to be removed to decrease the risk of infection or a very rare autoimmune condition called sympathetic ophthalmia, which can cause vision loss in the other, unaffected eye. Some patients may be born with congenital abnormalities requiring the use of a prosthetic eye. If cancer is detected in an eye or surrounding orbit, the treatment may involve removal of the affected eye to decrease the risk of cancer spreading to other parts of the body.

When Is an Ocular Prosthesis Placed? • After a natural eye is removed for any of the above reasons, the tissues in the orbit need time to heal and become strong enough to hold the prosthetic shell over the implant. Once the tissues heal well over the implant and if there is no exposure of the implant, then you may have an overlying prosthetic shell custom fitted. This usually occurs about 6 weeks after the implant is surgically placed.

Living with an Ocular Prosthesis • After the shell has been fitted, very little maintenance is necessary. Clean your prosthetic shell approximately once a week as directed by your eye doctor. This should help maintain longer-term fit and preservation. Your eye doctor will examine the eye socket periodically to make sure that the tissues over the implant remain healed. The prosthetic shell should be polished by an ocularist once a year. In most cases, patients are very satisfied with the appearance and comfort of their ocular prostheses.

Additional Resources

https://ocularist.org/resources_faqs.asp/
https://eyewiki.aao.org/Enucleation18

18 · Systemic Diseases That Affect Vision and the Eye

Diabetes Mellitus

MICHELLE SY GO, MS, MD

What Is It? • Diabetes mellitus is a systemic condition that is associated with abnormal sugar levels in the bloodstream. The body normally produces the hormone insulin to regulate the amount of sugar in the bloodstream. However, in diabetes, the body either does not produce appropriate amounts of insulin, as in type 1 diabetes, or it becomes resistant to the effects of insulin, as in type 2 diabetes. Both of these problems may cause high blood sugar, which can result in serious damage to blood vessels and the organs they supply. The eye is one of the first places in the body to be affected by diabetes. Diabetic retinopathy (or damage to the retina from diabetes) is the leading cause of vision loss in working-age adults in the United States.

Symptoms: What You May Experience • Diabetes can affect the eyes in many ways. You may notice blurry or fluctuating vision related to swelling in the cornea, lens, and retina. Diabetes also increases the chance of having cataracts, which can cause decreased vision and glare. Some people with severe diabetic retinopathy may have vision loss due to bleeding within the eye (vitreous hemorrhage), detachment of the retina, or very high eye pressure from scarring of the eye's drainage system (neovascular glaucoma).

Examination Findings: What the Doctor Looks For • An eye exam may reveal changes in vision that require a new glasses prescription due to swelling of the lens with high blood sugar levels. Your eye doctor will also look for cataracts as well as bleeding or swelling in the retina. They will also check carefully for abnormal blood vessel growth in the front or back of the eye, which is a sign of more advanced disease called proliferative diabetic retinopathy. Special photos and scans of the eye may be required to fully evaluate your eye disease.

What You Can Do • Good blood sugar control may slow down the damage caused by diabetes. It is important to work closely with your primary care doctor to optimize your blood sugar, blood pressure, and cholesterol. Routine laboratory testing and blood glucose monitoring may help your doctors determine how well your blood sugars are being controlled. Diet and exercise are helpful in improving insulin resistance in type 2 diabetes. You may also need to take medications or insulin to control your blood sugar. If you smoke, it is highly encouraged that you quit as smoking may cause damage to various parts of the body, including the blood vessels.

When to Call the Doctor • The American Diabetes Association recommends that patients with type 1 diabetes get an eye exam within the first 5 years of diagnosis and that those with type 2 diabetes get one soon after they are diagnosed. Annual eye exams are recommended, sometimes even more frequently if abnormalities are seen. You should also call the eye doctor if you are experiencing changes in vision, loss of vision, eye pain, flashing lights, or new floaters.

Treatment • The most important treatment is to get your blood sugar under control. This may require a combination of lifestyle changes and medications. Prevention is key. Eye-specific treatments vary depending on how the diabetes is affecting your eyes. You may need routine eye exams or new glasses early in the course of retinopathy, but more serious eye and retinal complications will require several laser treatments, multiple repeated eye injections, and/or one or more eye surgeries.

Prognosis: Will I See Better? • Visual prognosis is related to the severity of diabetic changes already present in the eye. Most people with good control of their diabetes retain good vision. Changes that are caught earlier have a better chance of successful treatment. Once irreversible damage occurs to the retina or optic nerve, the prognosis becomes worse. There is no treatment available to open retinal blood vessels that have already closed as a result of high blood sugars. Visual recovery is often guarded after eye surgery for the consequences of diabetic retinopathy. This is why it is important to take care of your diabetes, blood pressure, and cholesterol and see your doctors regularly to help you prevent certain complications of diabetes and to identify and treat those treatable abnormalities before the damage becomes irreversible.

Additional Resources

https://nei.nih.gov/health/diabetic/retinopathy

https://eyewiki.aao.org/Diabetic_Retinopathy

http://www.diabetes.org/

Hypertension (High Blood Pressure)

MICHELLE SY GO, MS, MD

What Is It? • High blood pressure, or hypertension, means that pressure in the arteries carrying blood to the body's organs is abnormally high. Excessively high blood pressure can damage important organs like the heart, brain, kidneys, and eyes. About 1 in 3 adults in the United States have hypertension. Most of the time there is no identifiable cause and the condition is called primary hypertension; in some cases, there is a known reason such as a hormone-releasing tumor or a narrowing of blood vessels leading to the kidneys.

A blood pressure reading is made up of two numbers in the form of the systolic pressure (during a heartbeat) over the diastolic pressure (in between heartbeats). A normal blood pressure is typically less than 120/80 mm Hg (mm Hg = millimeters of mercury). Current guidelines state that a repeatable blood pressure of 130/80 or higher suggests hypertension.

Symptoms: What You May Experience • Many people with hypertension have no symptoms and thus do not know that they have a potentially serious disease. When symptoms are present, it is usually due to very elevated or sudden episodes of hypertension. In these cases, blood pressure readings can be as high as 180/120 mm Hg or more. Symptoms include headaches, visual changes, and stroke-like symptoms such as confusion, difficulty speaking, or weakness on one side of the body. Hypertension can also cause injury to the heart leading to chest pain and difficulty breathing.

Examination Findings: What the Doctor Looks For • Abnormalities in the eye due to hypertension are best seen on a dilated eye exam. These include blood vessel changes, bleeding in the retina, leakage from blood vessels leading to retinal swelling, and damage to the nerve fibers in the retina. Sometimes veins in the eye may also get blocked from thickened arteries, resulting in a retinal vein occlusion. Severe hypertensive retinopathy may result in abnormal growth of new blood vessels, similar to proliferative diabetic retinopathy. There may also be a swollen optic nerve or changes in the choroid, which is a layer of blood vessels and connective tissue underneath the retina.

What You Can Do • The first step is to get your blood pressure checked. If it is consistently elevated, your primary care doctor will likely recommend lifestyle modifications such as changes in diet, limiting salt intake, exercise, and smoking cessation. If your blood pressure is higher, or does not respond to lifestyle modification alone, you may need to take medication to bring it under control.

When to Call the Doctor • You should undergo a routine eye exam if you have hypertension. Call your eye doctor's office if you have changes in vision or loss of vision. Go to the nearest emergency department if you are experiencing any of the previously mentioned symptoms of stroke or heart attack.

Treatment • The most important step is to work with your primary care doctor to bring the blood pressure under control. If you have abnormal blood vessel growth, blocked veins, or swelling in the retina that affects the central vision, it may be necessary to be treated with eye injections and/or laser therapy.

Prognosis: Will I See Better? • Long-term changes in the blood vessels of the eye can irreversibly damage important structures such as the retina and optic nerve. Visual prognosis is better for those who have only mild or acute changes from hypertension since these are more easily reversed.

Additional Resources

https://www.cdc.gov/bloodpressure/index.htm

http://eyewiki.aao.org/Hypertensive_retinopathy

Carotid Artery Disease (Ocular Ischemic Syndrome)

MICHELLE SY GO, MS, MD

What Is It? • Carotid artery disease is the general term for narrowing (stenosis) of the carotid artery or its branches. This is generally caused by atherosclerosis, or build-up of fatty plaque inside the blood vessel—the same process that can block arteries in the heart and cause a heart attack. Each person has a right and left common carotid artery that carries blood from the heart and runs up each side of the neck. Each common carotid artery splits into two branches to make the external and internal carotid arteries. The internal carotid arteries carry blood to the brain and eyes.

Poor blood flow through the carotid and/or internal carotid artery can lead to a rare condition called ocular ischemic syndrome. Ocular ischemic syndrome from atherosclerosis usually occurs in people older than 50 years of age, and is more common in men than in women. Other causes of ocular ischemic syndrome include multiple eye muscle surgeries, radiation to the neck, and inflammatory diseases such as temporal (giant cell) arteritis. The severity of ocular ischemic syndrome is affected by the degree of narrowing in the carotid circulation, and whether or not the body has developed alternate routes of blood flow to bypass the blockage and supply the eye.

Symptoms: What You May Experience • Some people may have no symptoms with carotid artery disease. The most serious complication is a stroke. Carotid artery disease can cause a "mini-stroke," also known as a transient ischemic attack (TIA). The symptoms of a TIA can be the same as in a stroke except that they are temporary, lasting only minutes or up to 24 hours. You may also experience sudden loss of vision in one eye, which can be temporary or permanent depending on how quickly blood flow can be restored. Other symptoms include new blind spots, difficulty distinguishing colors, eye pain, and light sensitivity. Vision loss may occur more slowly if ocular ischemia develops over a longer period of time.

Examination Findings: What the Doctor Looks For • The eye examination may reveal changes in the back of the eye including retinal blood vessel abnormalities, bleeding in the retina, optic nerve swelling, and abnormal blood vessel growth similar to that seen in proliferative diabetic retinopathy. Changes can also occur in the front of the eye, including corneal swelling, bleeding (hyphema), abnormal blood vessel growth, inflammation, and cataract. If abnormal blood vessels grow in the drainage system of the eye, the eye pressure may be high and cause glaucoma (neovascular glaucoma). Your eye doctor may also order additional testing such as a fluorescein angiogram, in which your retina is photographed after dye is injected into a vein.

What You Can Do • The risk factors for carotid artery disease are similar to those for heart disease. If you smoke, you should stop. You should follow regularly with a general physician to control your blood pressure, blood sugar, weight, and cholesterol.

When to Call the Doctor • You should call 911 if you have any symptoms of stroke or sudden loss of vision. Even if your symptoms are temporary, you should go to the emergency department right away to be evaluated. Do not drive yourself. Call your eye doctor for a routine eye examination if it has been longer than a year since your last check-up.

Treatment • If your eye doctor suspects that you have carotid artery disease or ocular ischemic syndrome, they may ask your primary care doctor to order an imaging test such as an ultrasound, magnetic resonance angiography (MRA), or computed tomography angiography (CTA) of the blood vessels in the neck. Knowing the amount of blockage in one or both carotid arteries is important in determining the next step. If the blockage is mild, the treatment is typically medical rather than surgical. This means that your primary care doctor is likely to start medications and work with you to make lifestyle changes to help control your risk factors for stroke. If you have severe blockage and you are healthy enough for surgery, you may benefit from a procedure that cleans out the blockage from the carotid artery (carotid endarterectomy). Some people cannot have this surgery but may still be considered for another procedure to help restore blood flow called carotid angioplasty and stenting, which is performed using a catheter inserted through a blood vessel in the groin.

Prognosis: Will I See Better? • Carotid artery disease and ocular ischemic syndrome can cause serious complications such as stroke and blindness. If caught and treated early enough, you may retain functional vision. However, studies have shown that about 40% people diagnosed with ocular ischemic syndrome die within 5 years of diagnosis. Therefore, it is extremely important to identify and manage your risk factors before you develop either of these diseases.

Additional Resources

https://www.nhlbi.nih.gov/health-topics/carotid-artery-disease
http://eyewiki.aao.org/Ocular_Ischemic_Syndrome

Multiple Sclerosis

MICHELLE SY GO, MS, MD

What Is It? • Multiple sclerosis (MS) is an inflammatory disease that damages the myelin sheath, a fatty outer coating of nerves in the brain and spinal cord. Damage to this outer coating in multiple sclerosis is called demyelination. MS typically affects young adults starting in their 20s and 30s and is about twice as common in women than men. The disease causes specific types of lesions, such as those in the optic nerve, spinal cord, and parts of the brain involving bowel and bladder function. The two broad categories of MS are relapsing-remitting and progressive disease. Relapsing-remitting MS is the most common type and is characterized by stable disease in between flares, or episodes of worsening. Progressive disease means that there is continuous worsening that happens either at the beginning or after an initial period of relapsing-remitting disease. A clinically isolated syndrome is the term used when a single episode of demyelination occurs in a person without any history of MS.

Symptoms: What You May Experience • The most common symptom involving the eye is painful loss of vision from optic neuritis, which is inflammation of the optic nerve. Optic neuritis may lead to poor color vision, blind spots, blurry vision, and pain with eye movement. As many as 75% of people with MS develop optic neuritis at some point. Abnormal eye movements leading to double vision and an inability to move the eyes in certain directions are also quite common. The eyes can also involuntarily quiver and cause an unpleasant bouncing sensation called oscillopsia. Inflammation in the vitreous gel, located in the back of the eye, occurs rarely in MS but may lead to eye pain, eye redness, light sensitivity, blurry vision, retinal swelling, and floaters. Systemic symptoms may include abnormal sensation in the body, difficult movement, incoordination, extreme fatigue, bowel and bladder dysfunction, and vertigo.

Examination Findings: What the Doctor Looks For • Abnormalities related to optic neuritis include decreased visual acuity, difficulty distinguishing colors, blind spots in the visual field, and an abnormal pupil reaction. A swollen optic nerve head is only present on exam in one-third of people with optic neuritis. The exam may also reveal difficulty or pain when looking in a certain direction, slowed movement of one eye compared to the other, abnormal movement of the eyes, or misalignment of the two eyes. A dilated eye exam will be performed to look for inflammation in the vitreous gel. Your eye doctor may order a visual field test and take photos of the optic nerve. Sometimes a brain scan (usually an MRI) is needed to look for areas of inflammation in the brain and optic nerve.

What You Can Do • There is no way to prevent or cure multiple sclerosis. If you already have a diagnosis of multiple sclerosis, you should continue regular followups with your neurologist. Certain medications can reduce relapse rates and improve the time to recovery from an episode.

When to Call the Doctor • Tell your doctor about systemic symptoms that could represent a flare or infection. Call your eye doctor or go to the nearest emergency department if you have sudden double vision, pain with eye movement, and/or loss of vision. Gilenya (fingolimod), which is a disease-modifying agent used in MS, can cause swelling in the retina so it is important to have routine eye examinations before, during, and after it is used.

Treatment • Studies have shown that intravenous steroids can result in faster recovery during an episode of optic neuritis; however, they do not impact the long-term visual outcome compared to those who do not receive intravenous steroids. If you have double vision or abnormal eye movements that do not improve over time, you might benefit from prism glasses or eye muscle surgery. A neurologist may recommend systemic disease-modifying agents to help manage MS. Other medications are aimed at treating the symptoms of MS.

Prognosis: Will I See Better? • Most who experience optic neuritis for the first time will recover vision back to baseline, which may be 20/20 if they do not have any other eye problems, although full recovery may take up to one year. About 8% may have vision that is 20/40 or worse after the first episode. Multiple episodes of optic neuritis are associated with worse visual outcome. Most people with abnormal eye movements will also improve over the course of a few months to one year.

Additional Resources

https://www.nationalmssociety.org

https://eyewiki.aao.org/Demyelinating_Optic_Neuritis

Autoimmune Diseases

MICHELLE SY GO, MS, MD

What Is It? • Autoimmune diseases are a broad group of disorders wherein the body's immune system responds abnormally to its own cells and tissues. Over 50 million people in the United States suffer from auto-immune diseases such as systemic lupus erythematosus, rheumatoid arthritis, Sjögren syndrome, and Graves' disease, to name just a few. While the underlying cause of autoimmune conditions is unknown, there are likely many factors that contribute to disease development such as genetics, environment, and prior infections.

Symptoms: What You May Experience • Different tissues and organ systems can be affected depending on the kind of autoimmune disease. Some generalized symptoms you may experience include fatigue, joint pain and swelling, weight loss, fever that comes and goes, and abdominal pain. Eye-specific symptoms include eye pain, eye redness, foreign-body sensation, light sensitivity, decreased vision, changes in position of the eye or eyelid, and double vision.

Examination Findings: What the Doctor Looks For • For diseases that can cause inflammation around the eye, it is important to note the eyelid position as well as any bulging of the eyes or lacrimal glands. Your doctor may use a device called a Hertel exophthalmometer to measure protrusion of the eyes from the eye socket, which can occur in Graves' disease. Eye movements and alignment will be examined as well.

Autoimmune disease can also cause inflammation on the eye surface and within the eye. The eye may be dry, red, or tender, or have nodules or areas of thinning on its surface. There can be abnormal cells and protein in the fluid inside the eye. Inflammation can cause the iris to stick to other structures inside the eye such as the cornea and lens. Autoimmune diseases can cause high or low eye pressure. Involvement of the back of the eye includes inflammation and leakage of blood vessels in the retina, retinal swelling, optic nerve swelling, and debris or cells in the vitreous. There may be noticeable lesions in the retina or the layers behind the retina—the choroid and sclera. Your doctor may need to order additional imaging and laboratory testing.

What You Can Do • In general, most people who develop autoimmune disease cannot prevent their disease from occurring. The few exceptions include autoimmune diseases that have known associations with infections such as Lyme disease, as well as reactive arthritis, which has been linked to diarrheal and genitourinary infections. Even in cases of infection, it is challenging to predict who will develop autoimmune disease and who will not.

When to Call the Doctor • Call your eye doctor if you are experiencing a flare-up of a known autoimmune condition, a new infection, or any other unusual health symptoms. People who take anti-inflammatory medications to control autoimmune disease are more vulnerable to infections. Some medications such as steroids and Plaquenil (hydroxychloroquine) have side effects that involve the eye. You should have routine eye examinations to monitor these side effects.

Treatment • Your eye doctor will likely need to work together with your primary care doctor or rheumatologist to coordinate systemic and eye-specific treatments. Treatments for the whole body can include medications by mouth, injection, or intravenous infusion. Medications can be delivered locally to the eye with eye drops, eye injections, or implants. Sometimes, it is necessary to have eye surgery for treatment or to confirm a diagnosis of autoimmune eye disease with a biopsy.

Prognosis: Will I See Better? • Disease severity and ocular involvement can vary greatly among different individuals depending on the type of autoimmune disease. The goal is to control inflammation and stabilize disease early, before permanent damage occurs to important structures in the eye.

Additional Resources

https://www.aarda.org

https://www.womenshealth.gov/a-z-topics/autoimmune-diseases

Migraine

MICHELLE SY GO MS, MD

What Is It? • Migraine is a common headache syndrome related to dysfunctional firing of nerve clusters in the brain and upper neck. This disorder affects over 37 million Americans and tends to run in families. It is more common in women than men and occurs most often in adults aged 30–39 years old. The typical sequence of events during a migraine episode are prodrome, aura, headache, and postdrome. Most people will not experience an aura, and some people may not even have a headache (called an acephalgic migraine or migraine equivalent).

Symptoms: What You May Experience • Approximately 3 out of 4 people with migraines experience a prodrome about 1–2 days prior to developing a headache. Symptoms of prodrome include yawning, change in mood (either good, bad, or irritable), and craving certain foods. A quarter of people experience an aura, usually occurring with the headache. Visual auras may include shimmering lights, zigzag lines, crescent patterns, stars, blind spots, and even loss of vision. The visual aura develops over a few minutes to an hour and typically recovers first in the central visual field. Auras can also be new sounds, sensations, and movements, or the loss of these functions. The migraine headache is usually on one side and throbbing in nature. You may feel nauseated and bothered by light, noises, or smells during the headache, which may last a few hours to several days. After the headache, you may feel tired or have pain with rapid head movement as part of the postdrome.

Migraine can be confused with stroke especially when the aura occurs quickly, involves loss of function, occurs in older individuals, or when there is no accompanying headache. Differentiating between migraines, transient ischemic attack (TIA or "mini" stroke), or stroke can be particularly difficult in these cases.

Examination Findings: What the Doctor Looks For • The main reason to have your eyes checked in cases of migraine is to rule out other more serious conditions such as glaucoma, optic nerve disease, blockage of a retinal blood vessel, and stroke. With migraines, the eye examination is usually normal. However, abnormal examination findings during a migraine may include pupil abnormalities, misalignment of the eyes, and blind spots. These usually resolve with time.

What You Can Do • If you have a history of migraines, you may have identified certain triggers such as stress, irregular sleep patterns, menstrual cycle (for women), certain foods, caffeine, and alcohol. It is helpful to avoid triggers when possible.

When to Call the Doctor • If you notice any new visual symptoms, you should notify your eye doctor. As mentioned above, some migraine symptoms can mimic TIA and stroke. A new severe headache could be a sign of something more serious such as bleeding in the brain. You should call 911 if you feel that you are having the "worst headache of your life" or have symptoms of stroke.

Treatment • Aside from avoiding triggers, certain medications may be helpful in decreasing the number of migraine episodes and relieve symptoms. These include over-the-counter pain relievers, caffeine, and prescription medications. The newest class of medications for migraine are antibodics. Botox injections are also used to help certain individuals with migraines. Talk to your primary care physician or neurologist about which treatment is right for you.

Prognosis: Will I See Better? • The visual prognosis is very good for people with migraine. Full visual recovery is typical.

Additional Resources

https://eyewiki.org/Ophthalmologic_Manifestations_of_Migraines
https://www.aao.org/eye-health/diseases/what-is-migraine

Temporal (Giant Cell) Arteritis

MICHELLE SY GO, MS, MD

What Is It? • Temporal arteritis, also known as giant cell arteritis, is an inflammatory disease that damages medium and large blood vessels that carry blood to the eyes, brain, and other important organs in the body. Inflammation of blood vessels, called vasculitis, can even affect the aorta, which is a large vessel connected directly to the heart. It is extremely rare to get temporal arteritis before 50 years of age. Over 80% of people with temporal arteritis are over the age of 70. This disease is most common in people of Scandinavian and northern European descent. Women are affected more than men. The most feared outcome of this disease is permanent vision loss in both eyes.

Symptoms: What You May Experience • The classic symptoms of temporal arteritis are headache, severe jaw pain that is associated with chewing, scalp tenderness, unexplained weight loss, poor appetite, fatigue, and fever. Up to half of people may also have a disease called polymyalgia rheumatica, which can cause shoulder and hip pain and stiffness. Symptoms specific to the eye include temporary or permanent vision loss usually in one eye, new blind spots, and double vision.

Examination Findings: What the Doctor Looks For • If you do not have visual symptoms, you may have a normal eye exam. Your eye doctor will examine the temporal arteries that run along each side of your head at the temples. Tender, large, ropy, or stiff arteries are suggestive of temporal arteritis. Your doctor will also check your visual acuity, eye pressure, color vision, pupils, and visual field before dilating your eyes. The optic nerve and retina may show signs of poor blood flow such as paleness, areas of bleeding, or fluffy white spots. If you have double vision, you may have misaligned eyes or trouble moving your eyes in certain directions. The doctor may also order bloodwork and imaging tests to help narrow down the diagnosis; however, the only way to confirm the diagnosis of temporal arteritis is by taking a biopsy of the temporal artery.

What You Can Do • There is no way to prevent temporal arteritis.

When to Call the Doctor • If you suspect temporal arteritis and develop loss of vision or double vision, you should call your eye doctor immediately. Timing of treatment is very important so you should not wait to seek help. If you develop worsening of general symptoms such as body aches, fatigue, or fever, you should notify your primary care doctor. If you do not have a prior diagnosis but your doctor suspects you have temporal arteritis, you should begin and continue treatment until you can be evaluated by an eye doctor.

Treatment • The main treatment for temporal arteritis is steroids, either by mouth or given intravenously. After an initial high dose of steroids, the dose can be slowly decreased over several months. Once started, steroids should never be stopped suddenly. Medications such as methotrexate and Actemra (tocilizumab) can also be used to decrease the amount of steroid needed, especially in those who cannot tolerate steroids.

Prognosis: Will I See Better? • About 15–20% of people with temporal arteritis will develop some degree of permanent vision loss. About 25–50% of people who have lost vision in one eye will have loss of vision in the other eye within a week if temporal arteritis is not treated promptly. That is why it is so important to get evaluated and treated as soon as possible. Quick and adequate treatment can prevent worsening of the affected eye and vision loss in the other eye.

Additional Resources

https://www.nanosweb.org/files/Patient%20Brochures/English/Giant%20Cell
    %20Arteritis%202017.pdf

https://eyewiki.aao.org/Giant_Cell_Arteritis

Sexually Transmitted Diseases

MICHELLE SY GO, MS, MD

What Is It? • Sexually transmitted diseases (STDs) are caused by bacterial, viral, or parasitic infections that pass from one person to another through intimate physical contact. According to the Centers for Disease Control and Prevention (CDC), there are about 20 million new cases every year. Examples of STDs than can affect the eye include human immunodeficiency virus (HIV), syphilis, gonorrhea, chlamydia, molluscum, and human papilloma virus. Genital herpes is usually caused by HSV-2, whereas herpetic infections of the eye are usually caused by HSV-1.

Symptoms: What You May Experience • STD-related eye infections can cause a wide range of symptoms including decreased vision, eye redness, eye pain, foreign body sensation, itching, irritation, light sensitivity, and discharge. Some viruses like molluscum can cause lesions or growths on the eyelid or conjunctiva. Infections that involve the back of the eye can cause floaters, blind spots, and severe permanent vision loss.

Examination Findings: What the Doctor Looks For • A complete eye examination will be performed since any part of the eye could be affected.

Eyelid lesions, conjunctival appearance, type of discharge, and pattern of corneal involvement can suggest a particular type of infection. Fluid in the eye may harbor cells, debris, or organism particles, and a sample may be collected to determine the causative organism. More severe infections may cause retinal lesions, blood vessel damage, and optic nerve damage.

What You Can Do • Be informed about how each disease is spread. The risk of getting an STD is lowered by abstinence, using condoms, and getting tested regularly depending on your exposure. You should talk to your sexual partner(s) about safe sexual practices. Be aware that some diseases can also be spread through contaminated needles, contact with open lesions, and from mother to child during pregnancy and childbirth. Pregnant women should be tested and treated for STDs according to their obstetrician's recommendations.

When to Call the Doctor • If you think you have an STD, you should call your primary care doctor. Call an eye doctor if you develop any changes in vision or ocular symptoms.

Treatment • Prevention is the best treatment. Antibiotic or antiviral medications can control or cure certain sexually transmitted diseases. You may need eye-specific therapy such as eye washes, eye drops or ointments, and injection of medication into or around the eye. Rarely, surgery may be indicated.

Prognosis: Will I See Better? • Visual prognosis is best with early diagnosis and treatment. Some infections are more aggressive or insidious than others, and permanent and/or severe vision can occur if left untreated.

Additional Resources

https://www.cdc.gov/std/healthcomm/fact_sheets.htm

https://familydoctor.org/condition/sexually-transmitted-infections-stis

Brain Tumors

MICHELLE SY GO MS, MD

What Is It? • Tumors are collections of abnormal cells that do not respond to the normal signals which control growth. The two main types of brain tumors are primary, meaning that they arise from the brain and surrounding tissues, and metastatic, meaning that they begin in a different part of the body and then travel to the brain. About 79,000 people in the United States were estimated to be diagnosed with a primary brain tumor in 2018; even more are diagnosed with metastatic disease. Brain tumors can also be categorized as benign or malignant. Benign brain tumors stay in and around the brain, whereas malignant, or cancerous, tumors may spread to other parts of the body.

Symptoms: What You May Experience • Brain tumors can affect your eyes in various ways depending on their location. Tumors affecting the optic nerves and optic chiasm (the crossroads between the right and left optic nerves) can cause decreased vision and blind spots. The signals from the optic nerves run in specific paths from the front to the back of the brain. A tumor affecting any part of this pathway will cause a particular pattern of blind spots, typically in both eyes. A person might experience double vision, difficulty moving the eyes, abnormal shaking of the eyes, or droopy eyelid. A tumor may also affect how images are interpreted by the brain. In these cases, you may have trouble recognizing faces and objects or determining where something is in relation to their surroundings.

Examination Findings: What the Doctor Looks For • The presence of a brain tumor can affect the pupils, visual acuity, eye movements and alignment, and visual field. Your eye doctor will also dilate your pupils to examine the retina and optic nerve. In certain cases, the optic nerve may be swollen due to high pressure in the head from a large tumor. Sometimes, optic nerve swelling is the first sign that is noticed before a brain tumor is diagnosed.

What You Can Do • Tobacco use can lead to cancers that eventually spread to the brain. If you smoke or use tobacco, you should stop. Tell your primary care doctor about any family history of cancer; they will guide you toward the appropriate cancer-screening tests based on your age and risk factors. Some environmental exposures and history of chemotherapy or radiation treatment can increase the risk of developing certain types of cancers. You should talk to your primary care physician or oncologist about these specific risks.

When to Call the Doctor • Call your eye doctor if you have any changes in vision or concerning ocular symptoms. Brain tumors affecting the eyes should be actively monitored by an eye doctor, often a neuro-ophthalmologist who specializes in diseases of the eye and brain.

Treatment • Treatments are based on tumor type, size, and location. Your plan may include chemotherapy, radiation, surgery, and/or treatments aimed at reducing symptoms. Double vision or abnormal eye position can sometimes be improved with prism glasses or eye muscle surgery.

Prognosis: Will I See Better? • Prognosis depends on the specific type of tumor, location, and size. Larger tumors affecting the optic nerves, optic chiasm, and the visual pathways may result in worse vision. Smaller tumors that stay stable, do not invade other tissues, and respond well to therapy typically demonstrate a better visual prognosis.

Additional Resources

https://www.aans.org/Patients/Neurosurgical-Conditions-and-Treatments
/Brain-Tumors

http://braintumor.org/brain-tumor-information/brain-tumor-facts

https://www.cancer.org/cancer/brain-spinal-cord-tumors-adults.html

https://www.cancer.org/cancer/brain-spinal-cord-tumors-children.html

Stroke and Cranial Nerve Palsies

MICHELLE SY GO, MS, MD

What Is It? • A stroke occurs when brain cells die from lack of blood and oxygen, usually resulting from a blocked or ruptured artery. Stroke is the second leading cause of death in the world after heart disease. About 800,000 people in the United States suffer from stroke each year—an average of 1 stroke occurs every 40 seconds.

A stroke can affect any part of the brain including the cranial nerves that control eye movements, such as cranial nerves 3, 4, and 6. Cranial nerve 3 controls four eye muscles, lifts the eyelid, and causes the pupil to get smaller in response to light. Cranial nerves 4 and 6 each controls one eye muscle. When a cranial nerve is injured and the resulting eye muscle is weak, this is referred to as a cranial nerve palsy.

An important distinction to stroke is microvascular disease, which refers to compromised blood flow in small vessels. Microvascular disease is common in diabetes and can also cause a cranial nerve palsy, but this typically resolves over a few weeks to months.

Symptoms: What You May Experience • The main symptoms of stroke can include facial droop, weakness or numbness in one or both arms, and slurred or difficult speech. These symptoms and the action to take can be remembered by the mnemonic FAST: Face, Arm, Speech, Time to act fast and call 911. Other symptoms can include altered mental status, severe headache, loss of coordination, nausea and vomiting, blurry vision, and new blind spots. Symptoms of cranial nerve 3, 4, or 6 palsy include double vision, trouble moving the eyes, abnormal head position or tilt, droopy eyelid, and abnormal pupils. Rarely, a "stroke" that affects the main blood supply to the eye can lead to a retinal artery occlusion and result in sudden, severe, and permanent vision loss.

Examination Findings: What the Doctor Looks For • Cranial nerve 3 palsy may cause abnormal pupil reaction to light and a difference in size between the pupils. The affected eyelid may be droopy; the eye may not move well up, down, or toward the nose. This leads to the classic appearance of the eye pointing down and out compared to its normal position. The findings in a cranial nerve 4 palsy are more subtle. The doctor may need to use special maneuvers or glasses to make the diagnosis. A cranial nerve 6 palsy will cause difficulty moving the affected eye away from the nose. This can lead to a cross-eyed appearance. A stroke can also cause blind spots in the visual field that can be picked up by examination or by a formal visual field test.

What You Can Do • About 80% of strokes could have been prevented. You can decrease your chances of getting a stroke by controlling risk factors like high blood pressure, high cholesterol, and obesity. If you smoke, it is important to stop. If you have a disease that puts you at risk for stroke such as diabetes, atrial fibrillation, or sickle cell disease, you should continue to work with your primary care doctor or specialist to optimize your health. If you have already had a stroke, you may need to take medications and work with specialists to regain strength and function.

When to Call the Doctor • You should call 911 and seek emergency help if you have any symptoms of stroke as mentioned above. Call your eye doctor if you notice double vision, abnormalities of the pupil or eyelid, new blind spots, or sudden vision loss. If you experience double vision, take note if it goes away with only one eye open at a time. Double vision resulting from cranial nerve palsy is only present with both eyes open.

Treatment • Systemic treatment for acute stroke requires a team of experts and fast action. The treatment plan usually depends on the type of stroke and when the symptoms began. The goal is to restore adequate blood flow as quickly as possible to prevent further tissue injury and cell death. Once your life-threatening issues are stabilized, the ocular problems can be addressed. If double vision has only recently started, one eye can be patched or covered temporarily to relieve the double vision. Prism glasses or eye muscle surgery can be considered eventually if the double vision does not improve over time. Treatments for a droopy eyelid may include taping up the eyelid in the short term, special glasses with crutches (ptosis crutches) to help lift the eyelids, and eyelid surgery. While there is no treatment to recover blind spots caused by a stroke, visual rehabilitation specialists can help maximize the function of the remaining vision.

Prognosis: Will I See Better? • Recovery from stroke can be variable. Wait at least several months to see if eye movements and eyelid function will recover. If there is little to no improvement after this time, the chances of recovery are low. Blind spots typically do not resolve, although there can be some improvement depending on recovery of injured brain tissue.

Additional Resources

https://www.strokeassociation.org

http://www.nanosweb.org/files/Patient%20Brochures/English/Microvascular
  CranialNervePalsy_English.pdf

https://eyewiki.aao.org/Cranial_Nerve_4_Palsy

https://eyewiki.aao.org/Acquired_Oculomotor_Nerve_Palsy

https://eyewiki.aao.org/Abducens_nerve_palsy

Human Immunodeficiency Virus

MICHELLE SY GO, MS, MD

What Is It? • Human immunodeficiency virus (HIV) is a small particle that attacks the body's immune cells and makes the body vulnerable to infections and certain types of cancer. HIV can lead to Acquired Immune Deficiency Syndrome (AIDS), which is when the number of immune cells reaches a critically low number or when a person develops an illness known to occur in AIDS patients. These AIDS-defining illnesses include pneumocystis pneumonia, cytomegalovirus (CMV) retinitis, toxoplasma infection in the brain, and some types of lymphoma. Over 39,000 people were diagnosed with HIV in the United States in 2016. Among those newly diagnosed, 68% were homosexual and bisexual men, 23% were heterosexual, and 9% were intravenous drug users. Of the 1.1 million people living with HIV (2015 U.S. data), 1 in 7 is unaware that they are infected. HIV/AIDS continues to be a global problem, but advances in HIV therapy and global health policy have curbed the number of new cases in the United States, Sub-Saharan Africa, Asia, and the Caribbean.

Symptoms: What You May Experience • Some people may not have symptoms during the beginning of an HIV infection, while others may feel like they have the flu for a few days to weeks. After this initial period, there may be no symptoms for many years. When a person develops AIDS, they are typically quite symptomatic with fever, chills, sweats, swollen lymph nodes, poor appetite, and weight loss, and they are prone to acquiring new infections. The ocular symptoms of HIV/AIDS are typically due to other infections and illnesses that occur as a result of a weakened immune system. These include lesions on the eyelids and conjunctiva, eye pain, light sensitivity, decreased vision, flashes of light, and new floaters.

Examination Findings: What the Doctor Looks For • HIV can cause fluffy white spots in the retina due to small blood vessel injury. More severe findings are usually due to infections that occur as a result of HIV/AIDS such as CMV, toxoplasmosis, syphilis, and tuberculosis. Abnormalities on exam may include lesions on the eyelids, cornea, and retina. Sometimes, severe retinal involvement can lead to a retinal detachment.

What You Can Do • Be informed about the ways that HIV is transmitted. It can spread through infected blood and bodily fluids such as semen and vaginal secretions. It can also be spread from mother to child during pregnancy, childbirth, and breastfeeding. You can decrease your chances of getting HIV by practicing abstinence, avoiding unprotected sex with multiple partners, and not sharing needles. Studies show that circumcision decreases the risk for HIV infection in men by 60%.

When to Call the Doctor • If you feel you have been exposed to HIV or have any of the concerning symptoms mentioned above, you should call your primary care doctor. People who are at very high risk of infection may benefit from taking medications every day to help prevent infection; this is known as pre-exposure prophylaxis (PrEP). If you feel you have been exposed to HIV in the last 72 hours, talk to your doctor right away about post-exposure prophylaxis (PEP). Call your eye doctor if you develop loss of vision, eye pain, light sensitivity, or flashes and floaters.

Treatment • There is no cure for HIV/AIDS. Preventing infection is key. Once infected, treatment consists of highly active antiretroviral therapy (HAART). This combination treatment includes 3 or more medications that target the virus in multiple ways. Antibiotic medications are also necessary to help prevent serious infections when the immune system is weakened.

Prognosis: Will I See Better? • HAART has dramatically changed the prognosis for those living with HIV. About 81% of people on HAART will achieve viral suppression, meaning that HIV virus is not detectable in the blood. If you begin treatment early, you have a good chance of keeping your health and vision intact. Visual prognosis is typically poor if there are lesions involving the optic nerve or central retina (macula).

Additional Resources

https://www.cdc.gov/hiv/default.html

https://eyewiki.aao.org/Ocular_Involvement_in_HIV/AIDS

19 · Cosmetic Eyelid Surgery

ANNA GINTER, MD, KENNETH NEUFELD MD,

AND JULIE A. WOODWARD, MD

What Is It? • As time passes, our eyelids become droopy due to the natural aging process. The entire forehead and eyebrows can also droop, which emphasizes the droopy appearance of the eyelids. Tissues that were once firm become softer, allowing the natural fat surrounding the eyeballs to herniate, or bulge forward, thus creating "bags" under the eyes. These bags cast shadows on the thin, bony lower rim of the orbit, emphasizing dark circles under the eyes.

There are two types of wrinkles that affect the face and eyes. Dynamic wrinkles occur when we make facial expressions. An example of dynamic wrinkles are the crow's feet areas (at the outer corner of the eyes) that increase when we smile. These dynamic wrinkles are often caused by thickening that occurs with age of some of the eyelid and facial muscles surrounding the eyes. Thickened muscles in the lower eyelids look like little bags beneath the eyelashes, while thickened muscles in the forehead emphasize the vertical frown lines between the eyebrows. The wrinkles that are present when the face is still are called static wrinkles, and are caused by the breakdown of skin collagen due to sun damage.

While some tissues, such as the eyelid muscles, thicken with age, other tissues thin. The skin overlying the bony rim of the orbit surrounding each eye becomes thin, which adds to the appearance of dark circles under the eyes. Beneath this area is another area of skin thinning along a ligament in the cheek. This area delineates a second "bag," which lies between the lower eyelid and the cheek and is called a festoon.

The following procedures are examples of typical cosmetic oculoplastic surgeries designed to reduce the effects of aging on the eyelids. Oculoplastic surgery is a subspecialty field of ophthalmology that is concerned with both cosmetic and functional aspects of the eyes and surrounding facial structures.

Upper Eyelid Blepharoplasty • Blepharoplasty is the medical term for eyelid lift. The surgeon may use various instruments to perform blepharoplasty surgery, including a steel blade, a laser, or a heated cautery instrument. The laser and cautery are particularly useful for decreasing bleeding during the procedure. Regardless of the technique used, the results are similar. This outpatient surgery is typically performed in the operating room or minor operating room with sedation and locally injected numbing medication.

An upper eyelid blepharoplasty is a procedure to lift the tissues of the upper eyelid. First, an incision is made in the upper eyelid crease, where the resultant scar will remain hidden after surgery. The amount of drooping skin, muscle, and bulging fat in the upper eyelid is carefully measured by the ophthalmologist during surgery to determine how much can be removed above the eyelid crease, while ensuring that the patient can still comfortably close their eyes after surgery. The wound is stitched closed at the end of the procedure, and an antibiotic ointment is placed on the incision for about 7–10 days. The stitches are usually removed in the office one week after surgery. Risks of this procedure should be discussed with your surgeon.

Brow Lift • If the eyebrows sag downward because of age and gravity, they can be lifted in a surgery called a "brow" or "forehead" lift. This surgery can be combined with an upper eyelid blepharoplasty. There are two common methods for operating on sagging brows. In a direct brow lift, an incision is made along the top edge of each eyebrow or at the hairline and excess skin and muscle are removed. The eyebrows are then lifted when the incisions are closed with stitches. In an endoscopic brow lift, incisions are made in the hairline, where the scars will be less noticeable. A tiny camera on the end of a lighted wand is inserted into the hairline incisions and used to place stitches that lift the eyebrows upward. Risks of this procedure should be discussed with your surgeon.

Eyelash Growth and Lifts • As brows and lashes change, thinner and shorter areas can be strengthened and to some degree restored by medicated cosmetic products containing prostaglandins. In cases where the lashes of upper eyelids are pointing downward, change in the direction of eyelashes can be performed via a laser lash lift, hence enhancing the cosmetic appearance of eyes.

Lower Eyelid Blepharoplasty • Lower eyelid blepharoplasty is a procedure to remove bulging fat bags under the lower eyelids. Some surgeons perform the procedure, also called transcutaneous blepharoplasty, by removing the fat bags through the skin beneath the eyelashes. This requires skin stitches for the incision at the end of the procedure. Other surgeons approach the fat through the inside of the lower eyelid in a method called transconjunctival blepharoplasty, which does not require skin stitches.

Removing the lower eyelid fat bags can result in loose skin in this area in some patients. There are two commonly used techniques to tighten this loose skin during a lower eyelid blepharoplasty. In the first technique, typically used in transcutaneous blepharoplasty, the loose skin can be cut out just beneath the skin incision, taking care not to remove so much skin that the lower eyelid is pulled down and out of position. The second technique to tighten the loose skin is laser skin resurfacing. A specialized laser vaporizes the top layer of skin and causes the loose skin to contract. This technique can be used to minimize wrinkles on the entire face. As the skin heals after the laser resurfacing, you may be instructed to cleanse and moisturize the skin frequently and avoid makeup for at least 10 days following the procedure. Also, the resurfaced skin may remain slightly pink for 4–6 months after laser treatment, which may require camouflage makeup.

Botulinum Toxin (Botox) Injection • Botulinum toxin, or Botox, is a medication injected to paralyze muscles. Botulinum toxin injection, in which the medication is injected into certain muscles of the face, is a popular method of treating dynamic wrinkles. Typically, botulinum toxin is injected with a tiny needle into the facial muscles in the forehead and surrounding the eyes during an office visit. The medication usually requires several days to take effect and lasts for 3–4 months, after which the injections can be repeated. Long-term use can result in the need for fewer injections. Too-frequent use (multiple intervals of less than 30 days) can result in the rare production of antibodies, which leads to the medication no longer working.

Filler Injection • Injection of filler material is an option used primarily for static wrinkles. Two types of such filler material exist: (1) non-dissolvable (which are currently falling out of favor) and (2) dissolvable, based upon a "hyaluronic acid" molecule. Such injectables come in varying levels of thickness with different brands, suitable for varying volume augmentation purposes. Some are designed to fill superficial wrinkles (e.g., around the mouth and eyes), while others offer fuller volume (e.g., into cheeks and lips) for restoring a more youthful appearance. Most fillers come with numbing medication mixed into the product, alleviating or reducing the pain of injection; in order to further decrease the discomfort of injection, you may request numbing cream prior to the injection itself. The more common side effects of filler augmentation include bruising from injection, whereas very rare but seriously devastating complications such as blindness may occur (e.g., if filler mitigates via vessels from the skin into the vascular supply of the eye). Loss of vision in such cases is unfortunately often permanent—with only slight improvement via measures to immediately dissolve the filler. Hyaluronic acid-based fillers are not permanent, but slowly degrade over about 2 years. Volume augmentation maintenance, in such cases, requires filler injections 1–2 times per year, with some dissolution possible via hyaluronidase injection (to reshape as needed).

Additional Resource

https://www.asoprs.org/eye-and-brow-lift

20 · Living with Visual Impairment

Impact of Living with Visual Impairment

RENEE HALBERG, MSW, LCSW

Understanding Feelings • Vision loss happens to people of all ages. With vision loss, it is normal to experience feelings of sadness, anger, frustration, guilt, or fear. It is also common to feel a loss of independence and self-esteem and to be concerned about becoming a burden to loved ones. Family members also react to vision loss in different ways: denial, acceptance, withdrawal, overprotection, or avoidance. Often, it is not easy to admit to having these feelings. Try to remember that these feelings are not right or wrong.

People who lose some or all of their vision may enter a period of grieving. How you feel is typically influenced by the degree and stability of your vision loss, your age, your cultural and religious beliefs, and the type of support system you have.

Ways to Help • If you are a caregiver of someone with vision loss, it is important to be a good listener and to encourage independence and social interaction. Resist the urge to be overly sympathetic or protective. It is also helpful to understand what they can see and do. Remember that all people with vision loss do not see the same.

If you are the one who has vision loss, it may be difficult to talk about how your vision loss affects your family and friends. You may feel concerned that you are hurting the feelings of your caregiver or other family members. However, sharing information with your family and friends about how your vision loss affects your everyday life can make it easier for others to offer help. Try to have important conversations when all parties are calm; openly discussing how vision loss affects all of your lives can help you feel closer. When friends and family are not enough, consider attending a support group. There are numerous support groups for people with vision loss from all sorts of eye diseases. Joining a support group can help you to learn from others, feel connected to those who understand what you are experiencing, and lessen feelings of anxiety and loneliness. Support groups can also help you find solutions and gain new perspectives on living with vision loss. In this Internet age, it is easier than ever to contact others with eye disease and to share insights and experiences through support group websites.

If you or a friend or family member lives with vision loss, make the effort to explore available community resources. Virtually every county or city has government-sponsored services, most of which are free of charge for people with visual impairment. These services can include special libraries with large-print or recorded books, or help in finding and purchasing low-vision aids. Tax benefits for people with impaired vision also exist.

When to Ask for Professional Help • A low-vision specialist is a professional trained to help people with impaired vision perform their daily activities. If you visit a low-vision specialist in your community, they will demonstrate different visual aids and help you decide which ones will help you. These aids can include magnifiers (in glasses, handheld, on a stand, or electronic), computerized reading devices, and other tools to help you perform your daily tasks. Not all of these aids may suit your needs, but exploring them is a good first step to learning to make the most of any vision that you may have.

Some low-vision specialists are experts in visual rehabilitation. These professionals will often come to your home to help you set up a user-friendly environment that serves your visual needs, and they can help you learn special techniques to perform your daily activities more effectively and with less frustration.

It is not unusual to experience high and low moods when dealing with vision loss. When the low periods interfere with your ability to function and just won't go away, you may have depression. Other signs of depression are a loss of interest in pleasurable activities, significant weight loss or gain, inability to sleep or sleeping too much, social withdrawal, frequent crying spells, irritability, anxiety, feelings of hopelessness and helplessness, and difficulty concentrating. If you have depression, it is essential to get professional help from a skilled and licensed professional. You can ask your primary care doctor for a referral to a licensed clinical social worker, psychologist, psychiatric nurse, or psychiatrist. It is a life-threatening emergency if you or someone you know expresses suicidal thoughts and plans: Call 911 and go to or have the person taken to the nearest hospital for assessment and treatment.

Creative Ways to Deal with Stress • We need to take care of ourselves in order to live fulfilling lives. Think about what brings you joy, encourages laughter, or gives you a sense of peace. Take a walk, sign up for a dance or yoga class, learn to meditate, listen to your favorite music, or use aromatherapy. Perhaps you would like to plant flowers and herbs, sculpt with clay, or record your life story on tape for your family. Spend time with other people who have a positive attitude and a sense of humor, and you will realize that you are not alone as you live with visual impairment.

Additional Resources
http://www.preventblindness.org/
http://www.afb.org/
http://www.aerbvi.org/
http://www.lighthouse.org/
http://www.loc.gov/nls/

Low Vision Aids and Strategies to Maximize Functional Vision

FAY JOBE TRIPP, MS, OTR/L, CLVT, CDRS

If vision impairment makes it difficult to complete daily tasks, simple strategies and adaptive devices can help improve functional vision, even in cases where vision impairment might be severe or permanent. You can use these strategies and visual aids to maximize function and efficiency when performing activities of daily living (ADLs) and instrumental activities of daily living (IADLs), allowing for more independence and safety when performing tasks at home, work, or out in the community. It may be helpful to work with a low-vision specialist in ophthalmology, optometry, occupational therapy, or orientation and mobility.

Compensatory Strategies and Devices • Because vision impairment affects each person in their own unique way, each individual will require strategies specific to their own needs. Generally, however, optimizing lighting, decreasing glare, and increasing magnification can improve functional vision when central vision is impaired, particularly with near vision tasks such as reading, writing, and computer work.

LIGHTING Full-spectrum white light can decrease glare and increase contrast. Direct the light toward the area where you are attempting to perform a task. Some lights may be adjustable to cool, natural, or warm temperatures depending on your preference. Consider brighter lights for near work and have lights available on your desk and in other work areas. A cellphone flashlight app or an LED flashlight may be useful as portable light sources.

GLARE CONTROL AND CONTRAST ENHANCEMENT Various sun filters that fit over existing glasses may be used to control glare. Use a light-yellow tint inside or in lower-light environments, and a hazelnut or amber tint outside or in brighter lighting environments. Position yourself with your back toward the window to avoid glare from sunlight. You can also position the computer monitor or TV away from windows to avoid glare. Placing lighter objects against a dark background and inverting the colors on your phone or computer monitor, so that the background is dark instead of light, can help increase contrast.

MAGNIFICATION Larger screens for your TV, computer, or smartphone may help you see text and pictures more easily. A handheld or standing magnifier with a light can be used to improve the view of small objects. Electronic video magnifiers or a closed circuit TV system may be useful for reading text or performing fine tasks. Smartphone apps and tablets often have the ability to enhance the magnification and contrast of text or other objects on the screen. Portable electronic magnifiers and desk electronic video magnifiers may help with reading, writing, and other near tasks. Handheld binoculars or a monocular telescope can be used to view objects that are far away; some telescopes can even be mounted on a pair of glasses. Wearable electronic glasses can also be used to enhance the view of your surroundings.

READING STRATEGIES Brighter lighting directed toward your reading material may help enhance contrast. Magnifiers, either handheld or electronic, may be used to enlarge text. Some electronic reading devices may also allow you to invert contrast. Use a line guide or solid color bookmark as you read to minimize visual clutter. If you have

double vision, block one eye temporarily with a patch or vision oc-
cluder, alternating eyes as appropriate. Audiobooks and podcasts are
available on many electronic tablets as an alternative.

Functional Mobility and Fall Prevention • Visual impairment can directly
affect mobility safety and community accessibility and also increases the
risk of falls. Common challenges may include decreased acuity in one or
both eyes, impaired depth perception, decreased peripheral vision, and
decreased functional vision related to glare. When visual impairment
is combined with physical limitations, there is an even greater increase
in the risk of falling. Physical limitations may include impaired muscle
strength, decreased joint range of motion, poor endurance, decreased
balance, and decreased sensation. If needed for walking, use of a mobility
aid like a sight cane or walker offers helpful sensory feedback for changes
in landscape or way-finding patterns. Prior to obtaining a mobility aid,
get professional guidance from a physical or occupational therapist to
ensure that you choose the best device. If you have significant visual limitations, a certified orientation and mobility specialist (coms) can provide instruction on how to use a mobility aid combined with strategies
to compensate for the vision impairment. Some types of aids, known as
durable medical equipment (dme), may be covered under insurance but
may require assistance of an Assistive Technology Professional (atp) for
assessment and training. The following strategies may help reduce the
risk of falling:

- Add lighting to dark areas to brighten your path.
- Use glare control in bright light or outdoor areas.
- Wear sensible, supportive, and non-slip shoes.
- Use a mobility aid or sight cane for added sensory input or physical
  stability.

For stairways:

- Use good lighting and glare control strategies.
- Hold the handrails.
- Use your feet for sensory input for height and depth perception.
- Add contrast color or reflective strips at the edge of steps.
- Avoid stairs if the risk is too high and instead use a ramp or elevator.

Driving Safety, Strategies, and Modifications • A common measure of independence is the ability to drive yourself. Even with normal vision, driving can be a challenge, but vision is not the only consideration for safety. There are vision requirements to obtain and keep your driver's license. Your state's Department of Motor Vehicle (DMV) Medical Review Board may require completion of a vision specialist form. They may also require that a comprehensive clinical assessment including vision, cognition, and physical skills be completed by an occupational therapist with specialized training in driving skill assessment (Certified Driver Rehabilitation Specialist, or DCRS). Common visual impairments that may cause driving challenges include decreased distance vision, poor night vision, decreased glare tolerance, loss of depth perception, and compromised peripheral vision. These visual changes may significantly impact driving safety and require self-restriction, vehicle modification, or delegation to another licensed driver. Your state DMV may also place restrictions on your license based on specific state driving requirements. The following strategies may be helpful:

- Compensate for decreased peripheral vision:
  — Perform head-turn scanning maneuvers.
  — Apply expanded-view mirrors to the existing side-view mirrors.
  — Apply a panoramic-view mirror on the existing rear-view mirror.
- Use glare-control sunglasses for brighter conditions during daylight hours, or at night for headlight glare control.
- Self-restrict driving when there are intermittent vision changes: delegate driving at night, on interstate highways, or during high-fatigue periods.
- Use a GPS system to assist with directions.
- Choose available safety features on automobiles: sensors with forward collision warning, rear cross-traffic alert, lane-departure warning, blind-spot warning, and parking assistance, among others.
- For vision that is stable but does not meet your state's DMV driving requirements, a bioptic telescope lens system to enhance distance vision may be allowed.

Additional Resources

Eschenbach Optik: https://www.eschenbach.com/

Independent Living Aids, Inc.: http://www.independentliving.com/

Maxi-Aids Low Vision: https://www.maxiaids.com/

Ocutech Telescope:s https://ocutech.com/

Optelec Low Vision: https://us.optelec.com/

Retinal Prosthesis (Argus II, the "Bionic Eye")

ANTHONY THERATTIL, BS AND LEJLA VAJZOVIC, MD

What Is It? • Much like a prosthetic arm or leg, the retinal prosthesis, or "Bionic Eye" was made to replace a part of the body that no longer works or is lost—in this case that part is the retina of the eye (see chapter 1 for a basic overview of the retina).

The retinal prosthesis is made by Second Sight under the name Argus II (the second generation of this technology) and is made of three main parts: glasses with a small camera, a small device the patient carries around which is essentially a tiny computer, and a band that encircles the outside of the eye and holds a very small electrode that is positioned within the eye via a surgical procedure. All three components communicate with each other to turn visual images from the camera into gradient lights that a blind patient can actually see, allowing them to interpret objects in space.

Who Needs a Retinal Prosthesis? • Patients with diseases that involve retinal degeneration could potentially benefit from a retinal prosthesis (see chapter 9 for an overview of retinal degeneration). These patients have slowly dying retinas that can't process light as well, causing gradually worsening vision over time that can progress to blindness. The Argus II is a Federal Drug Administration (FDA)–approved technology in the United States, Europe, and parts of Asia and can be used as an option for certain adult patients with end-stage retinitis pigmentosa (a specific type of retinal degeneration).

How Does It Work? • The retina normally receives light from a person's surroundings, turns that light into an electrical signal, and sends it to the brain where it is translated into shapes, colors, and movements, allowing us to see everything around us. The retinal prosthesis helps the damaged retina complete this process. The camera takes video of the surroundings and sends it to the computer where the image is converted into a unique electrical code. This code is sent to the electrode inside the eye, where the electrode stimulates a small part of the retina that can function with some help. The retina then relays this signal to the brain where the signal is processed to create an image that the patient sees.

What can a person see with a retinal prosthesis? Patients with a retinal prosthesis can see outlines and shapes of moving objects/people, surroundings with large contrast, and sometimes colors. People who use the prosthesis say that they can identify paved walkways, perceive doorway entrances, use lights for orientation and identify whether something is in front of them, among other things. Although they still can't see normally, this can be a significant change for a person who was previously blind. This new way of seeing can improve quality of life by providing more independence, better mobility, and greater comfort in social situations.

How Do I Learn More? • You can speak with your retina specialist about retinal prostheses and can also visit the Second Sight webpage for more information. These resources may help outline whether one meets the basic requirements to be eligible for the retinal prosthesis. If eligible, you can connect with experts who can answer additional questions and discuss whether the prosthesis is ultimately a good option.

What Is the Process Like? • Retinal prostheses are attached to the eye with surgery at certain regional hospitals where experienced retinal surgeons perform the surgery and the rest of the eye-care team continues treating the patient. After the surgery is performed, the patient's eye is given about 4 weeks to heal from the surgery. It is only after that when the patient's prosthesis device will be turned on and the settings adjusted specifically for them. From there, rehabilitation specialists will work with the patient so that they can learn to use the prosthesis to achieve their goals.

Routine yearly follow-up examinations are recommended for these patients to adjust their prosthesis settings and to examine ocular structures. As with any implantation of foreign material in the body, the biggest risk is infection. With time, the external portion of the prosthesis can become exposed to the environment and then infected. Therefore, it is important to continue follow-up examinations. Overall, the cost of the implant and surgery is around $150,000 and some health insurances will cover the cost in pre-approved individuals. The lifespan of the retinal prosthesis is unknown at this time. There are some individuals who have had it in their eye for over a decade and are still using the implant and functioning well with it.

Optical Coherence Tomography

S. TAMMY HSU, MD

Optical coherence tomography (OCT) is a rapid, non-invasive, non-contact imaging test that takes cross-sectional images of the various parts of the eye, most commonly the retina. This imaging technology works in a method similar to that of ultrasound, except it uses light waves instead of sound waves. There are no x-rays and no radiation. OCT is very safe with no known risks to the eye. OCT may show subtle signs of eye conditions that may otherwise not be easily seen by your eye doctor during a dilated eye examination. OCT is widely used to evaluate and monitor conditions such as age-related macular degeneration and diabetic macular edema. OCT can also be used to measure the retinal nerve fiber layer of the eye to assess the health of the optic nerve in glaucoma or suspected glaucoma.

The OCT testing can be done with or without dilating your pupil.

During OCT imaging, the ophthalmic photographer or ophthalmic technician will ask you to position your head so that your chin rests on the chinrest and your forehead rests against the forehead bar of the OCT machine. The photographer or technician may then ask you to look at a certain green target inside the OCT machine. If your vision is too blurry to see the target, that is okay since the photographer knows where to take the OCT picture based on the information provided by your eye doctor. The photographer or technician will then begin taking OCT pictures or "scanning" the part of the eye that your eye doctor requested, often your retina and/or optic nerve. The light in the machine is sometimes bright. During the testing, nothing will actually touch your eye. The testing may take anywhere from just a few minutes to 15 minutes depending on the number of scans requested by your eye doctor. No special precautions are needed after testing.

Additional Resources

https://www.aao.org/eye-health/treatments/what-is-optical-coherence-tomography
https://www.aao.org/eye-health/treatments/what-does-optical-coherence
-tomography-diagnose

Fundus Autofluorescence

MELISSA MEI-HSIA CHAN, MBBS

Fundus autofluorescence is an imaging technique used to evaluate the health of the retina and the underlying support tissue, called the retinal pigment epithelium (RPE). This imaging method highlights a substance called lipofuscin, which is a waste product that accumulates in the retina with age and is commonly referred to as the "wear-and-tear" pigment. Normally, light-sensing cells in the retina continually renew and the outer layers of these cells are shed and broken down into lipofuscin. Excessive lipofuscin accumulation can result in abnormal function and even death of the RPE cells, ultimately leading to visual impairment. Fundus autofluorescence may be useful for identifying damaged and dead cells in conditions such as age-related macular degeneration or other inherited retinal degenerations.

The imaging process is non-invasive and takes just a few minutes to complete. You will be asked to sit in front of a machine and rest your forehead on the headrest. You will then be asked to focus on a target in the machine while the photographer scans your retina.

Fluorescein Angiography

MICHAEL P. KELLY, FOPS

Fluorescein angiography is a diagnostic procedure in which images of the retina are taken using a specialized camera in a rapid sequence after a small amount of dye is injected into a vein in your arm or hand. The dye quickly flows to the blood vessels in the back of the eye (retina) and can highlight areas not receiving adequate blood flow or identify abnormal blood vessels not easily seen during a regular eye exam. This procedure is helpful in the evaluation of many retinal disorders including diabetic retinopathy, macular degeneration, and vascular occlusions. Although most often used to image the retina, fluorescein angiography can also be helpful in the evaluation of the iris and sclera.

Before the procedure, your eyes will usually be dilated with eye drops. Once fully dilated, your chin and forehead will be positioned so that your eyes are placed in front of a specialized camera, and several images of both eyes will be taken. The fluorescein dye will then be injected into a vein in your arm or hand, and at the same time, a series of images will be taken over the course of about one minute to record the dye as it flows through the retinal blood vessels. More images will be taken of both eyes at several intervals for the next 5–10 minutes, with opportunity for short rests in between. No x-rays are used.

There are some common side effects and reactions to the contrast dye. Your urine, sweat, and skin may appear slightly reddish-orange for up to 36 hours. You may also notice a temporary metallic taste in your mouth that lasts for several hours. Nausea and sometimes vomiting may also occur in about 5% of patients; it occurs about a minute after the dye has been given and lasts for only about 2 minutes. More rare but serious reactions can include hives and itching, swelling of the airway, anaphylaxis (systemic allergic reaction), and cardiac arrest. Because it is unknown if there are risks to the unborn fetus, most eye doctors delay performing fluorescein angiography in pregnant patients unless absolutely necessary. Fluorescein dye can cross into breast milk; therefore, planning ahead to express and store breast milk for feedings for at least 8–12 hours after the fluorescein angiogram should be considered. If you are scheduled for blood tests in the days following fluorescein angiography, inform your physician since fluorescein dye can interfere with some types of lab work.

Additional Resources

https://eyewiki.aao.org/Fluorescein_Angiography
https://www.aao.org/eye-health/treatments/what-is-fluorescein-angiography

Indocyanine Green Angiography

MICHAEL P. KELLY, FOPS

Indocyanine green angiography (ICGA) is very similar to fluorescein angiography in the way it is performed but is different in that it uses a different contrast dye called indocyanine green. This dye, when paired with a near-infrared camera, allows for more detailed imaging of the blood vessels *behind* the retina. While fluorescein angiography allows us to image the retina, ICGA allows us to look *through* the retina to image the choroid. Sometimes both fluorescein angiography and ICGA may be needed by the eye doctor on the same visit. ICGA can be helpful in identifying abnormal blood vessels that originate in the choroid and is useful in a variety of disorders including subretinal hemorrhage, pigment epithelial detachment, polypoidal choroidal vasculopathy, retinal angiomatous proliferation, central serous retinopathy, uveitis, and intraocular tumors. Reactions to indocyanine green dye are rare and include nausea (and sometimes vomiting), itching, and hives. You should avoid ICGA if you have a history of iodine allergy or previous adverse reaction to ICG dye. You should also avoid ICGA if you are or may be pregnant. Additionally, the results of some other lab studies, such as radioactive iodine uptake, may be affected if performed after ICGA.

Optical Coherence Tomography Angiography (OCT-A) Tomography

S. TAMMY HSU, MD

Optical coherence tomography (OCT) angiography, also known as OCT-A, is a commercially available non-invasive imaging method that uses the same technology as OCT to take hundreds of cross-sectional images. Advanced software is then used to create a detailed 3D map of the blood flow in the retina. These images can be directly compared with traditional OCT images, allowing the doctor to identify abnormal blood flow in different layers of the retina. This may be useful to assess early signs of retinal diseases that involve the blood vessels, such as diabetic retinopathy and macular degeneration.

During the imaging process, you will be asked to look at a fixed target in the OCT-A machine. The machine is non-contact and the entire process takes only a few minutes for each image. The total time spent depends on the number of pictures ordered, the region of interest, eye movement, and degree of cooperation.

Unlike fluorescein angiography, OCT-A is non-invasive (no needles or contrast dye needed). However, certain OCT-A machines may have a smaller field of view and not be able to detect leaking blood vessels or view the dynamic flow of contrast dye over time, which can be detected on fluorescein angiography. In some cases, your eye doctor may order both OCT-A and fluorescein angiography as part of a comprehensive eye evaluation.

Specialized Tests: Electroretinography, Electrooculography, and Visual Evoked Potential

ALESSANDRO IANNACCONE, MD, MS, FARVO

What Is Electroretinography (ERG)? • The ERG is a non-invasive objective test that measures the electrical activity of the retina. After adjusting to darkness, tiny contact lens–like or thread-like sensors are placed on the eye to sense electrical activity in response to light. The flash ERG is very similar to the "stress EKG" that is done to see how the heart responds when challenged. Flashes of light of varying brightness and speed are displayed, and the whole retina responds at once, generating an electrical impulse at each flash. This informs the eye doctor about the health of the retina.

Patients with retinitis pigmentosa will usually show reduced nighttime (rod) responses and variable reduction of daytime (cone) responses. Patients with earlier-onset retinal dysfunction, such as those with Leber's congenital amaurosis, will usually show very small or completely non-recordable responses early on. Macular dystrophies may show a mix of reduced daytime and nighttime responses. A flash ERG can also be performed on a sedated or fully asleep person in the operating room, if necessary, which may be helpful when evaluating a very young child with a suspected inherited retinal condition.

What Is Electrooculography (EOG)? • The EOG is a non-invasive test that measures the function of the retinal pigment epithelium (RPE), a specialized layer of cells underneath the retina. The RPE is important for keeping the retina healthy. The EOG is similar to a "resting EKG of the heart" with no special challenge and simply measures the change in the spontaneous flow of electricity coming out of the eye in dark and steady light conditions. This test is helpful in confirming the diagnosis of a unique macular dystrophy called Best disease. However, the EOG may also be abnormal in other related conditions affecting the same gene.

What Is Visual Evoked Potential (VEP)? • The optic nerve carries electrical signals from the retina toward the part of the brain known as the visual cortex. The function of the optic nerve can be measured with a special test called the VEP (visual evoked potential). This test involves placing a small metal disc (an "electrode") on the back of the head where the visual cortex is located, then measuring electrical signals when certain patterns of light are displayed. The most informative type of VEP is measured in response to a moving checkerboard pattern. The size, shape, and most importantly the timing (speed) with which visual information travels from the eye to the brain is recorded, and this information serves as a reliable health assessment of the optic nerves and optic pathways.

Ultrasound of the Eye

CATHY DIBERNARDO, RN

Ocular ultrasound, like other types of ultrasound, uses sound waves to look at ocular structures. It is quick, painless, and performed routinely in clinic. There are several different types of ultrasound that can be used to evaluate the eye.

BIOMETRY (ALSO KNOWN AS AXIAL LENGTH MEASUREMENT) This type of ultrasound is done prior to cataract surgery to measure the length of the eye and helps the surgeon determine the correct power of the artificial lens to be placed in your eye during surgery after the cataract is removed. The test is accurate and relatively simple. The eyes are first numbed using anesthetic eye drops, then a small fluid-filled cup is placed beneath the eyelids. A small probe is placed in the fluid, and the distance from the corneal surface (front of the eye) to the retina (back of the eye) is measured. These measurements help determine the intraocular lens power to allow the best-possible vision in the eye following cataract surgery.

ULTRASOUND BIOMICROSCOPY (UBM) Using very high ultrasound frequencies (40–100 MHz), the front portion of the eye (cornea, anterior chamber, iris, ciliary body, peripheral choroid, and even the conjunctiva) can be evaluated. The eyes are numbed using a topical anesthetic and a small probe surrounded by a fluid-filled balloon then touches the surface of the eye. The images obtained are very detailed and provide your surgeon with useful information about many different eye conditions such as corneal scaring, conjunctival growths, iris lesions, glaucoma, and ciliary body lesions or tumors.

CONTACT B-SCAN AND STANDARDIZED A-SCAN Typically, when you go to the eye doctor, your pupils will be dilated with eye drops, allowing the eye doctor to get an unobstructed view of the structures inside the eye. Occasionally, conditions exist that may prevent the eye doctor from getting a good look inside the eye. In these cases, they may order an ultrasound to help visualize eye structures behind that obstruction.

The eyes are numbed with anesthetic drops, and various probes that transmit sound waves are placed directly on the surface of eye or eyelids. A gel is used on the surface of the probe to aid in transmission of sound waves. You may be asked to look in different directions and the probes may be gently moved to various positions to obtain information that will be useful for your doctor.

B-scan provides two-dimensional images of areas inside the eye, while standardized A-scan provides one-dimensional images of spikes along a baseline. The tests are useful both individually and when used together for certain conditions. Some indications for B-scan and standardized A-scan include corneal opacities, dense cataracts, blood in the front or back of the eye, inflammation in the eye, retinal tears, retinal detachments, and tumors and other lesions. These types of ultrasound can also be used to evaluate the structures around the eye such as the eye muscles, optic nerve, and orbital (eye socket) tissue.

Appendix

How to Put in Eye Drops

WILLIAM L. RAYNOR, BS

Eye drops are vital to the management of a variety of eye-related conditions ranging from infection to glaucoma. However, there are many ways in which eye drops can be improperly administered, which may lead to ineffective treatment. That is why it is important to follow a few basic steps to ensure that eye drops are administered in a clean and effective manner.

Step 1: Wash your hands thoroughly with soap and water prior to touching your medication or your eyes.

Step 2: Some eye drop medications may require you to shake before use. Check the instructions listed on the eye drop bottle label to see if they specify whether shaking is necessary.

Step 3: Remove the cap from your eyedrop bottle and avoid touching the dropper tip to any surfaces throughout this entire procedure. Be sure to check the tip for any signs of contamination before proceeding.

Step 4: Tilt your head back so your face is pointing upward. This will make your eyes an easier target for the eye drop to fall in.

Step 5: Using your index finger, gently pull down on your lower eyelid to create a small pocket between your eye and eyelid.

Step 6: With the other hand, bring the bottle tip over your eye and squeeze one drop into the small pocket you have created with your lower eyelid. Check if your eye drop can be refrigerated. If the eye drop is cold, then you may be able to feel it more easily when it lands on the surface of your eye. Remember not to let the tip touch your eye or eyelids to minimize contamination and avoid eye injury.

Step 7: Lightly close your eyes and, using your index finger, apply gentle pressure to the inside corner of your upper and lower eyelids for 30 seconds. This allows the medication to be better absorbed by your eye instead of being drained away through your tear duct.

Step 8: Gently dab away any excess eye drop medication with a clean tissue. Be sure not to wipe as it may cause skin irritation.

Step 9: If the treatment regimen ordered by your doctor requires more than one drop per eye at a given time, wait at least 5 minutes in between eye drops to allow each medication to be fully absorbed by the eye.

Step 10: Replace the dropper cap, store your eye drop bottle in a safe and clean location, and wash your hands.

If you are having difficulty putting in your eye drops, then consider asking a family member or a friend for assistance. Consult your pharmacist or eye doctor with any questions.

Additional Resource

https://www.aao.org/eye-health/treatments/how-to-put-in-eye-drops

Glossary

abscess collection of pus

accommodation a slight change in the shape of the natural lens that allows one to see nearby objects

achromatopsia a retinal disease in which no colors are seen

Acquired Immune Deficiency Syndrome (AIDS) an infectious disease that weakens the body's immune system

acute hydrops a painful episode of corneal swelling usually seen in keratoconus

"after cataract" (posterior capsular opacity) a film that forms behind a lens implant

age-related macular degeneration a disease of older people that affects the center of the retina (macula)

amblyopia (lazy eye) decreased vision in one or both eyes that is caused by any of a variety of disruptions of normal visual development

anterior chamber the space inside the eyeball between the cornea and the front of the iris

aqueous humor the clear fluid that fills the anterior chamber of the eye

astigmatism an irregular curvature of the surface of the cornea

atrophy permanent loss of the use of a part of the body

autoimmune involving a malfunction of the body's immune system

basal cell carcinoma a type of skin cancer

benign noncancerous

black eye (orbital ecchymosis) a collection of fluid and blood in the tissues around the eye

blepharitis inflammation of the eyelid margins

blepharoplasty surgery to lift the eyelids

blepharospasm uncontrolled twitching of the muscles in the eyelids and around the eyes

blue-yellow color deficiency an inherited difficulty in distinguishing between the colors blue and

yellow botulinum toxin (Botox) a medicine injected into muscles to paralyze them

brow lift surgery to lift the eyebrows

Bruch's membrane a layer of tissue that separates the retina and retinal pigment epithelium from the choroid

capsular bag the natural bag that holds a lens or lens implant in place in the pupil of the eye

carcinoma a type of cancer

carotid artery disease narrowing of the carotid artery or its branches

cataract a clouding of the normally clear lens inside the eye

cellophane retinopathy (epiretinal membrane, macular pucker, preretinal gliosis) a thin sheet of abnormal scar tissue that grows over the retina

central nervous system the brain, the spinal cord, and their nerves

central retinal artery the blood vessel that supplies most of the retina

central retinal vein the blood vessel that drains most of the retina

central serous chorioretinopathy a disease in which fluid collects under the macula

cerebrospinal fluid (CSF) fluid that surrounds the brain, spinal cord, and optic nerves

chalazion a nodule of inflammation that forms a bump in the eyelid

choroid a blood vessel layer located between the retina and sclera

choroidal neovascularization (CNV) a patch of abnormal blood vessels and scar tissue that grows under the retina

ciliary body the part of the eyeball that produces aqueous humor

color blindness a deficiency in the way color is seen

computed tomography scan (CT scan) a specialized x-ray technique

cone a type of photoreceptor that processes colors and finely detailed images

congenital present at birth

conjunctiva the outer, clear tissue layer that covers the white part of the eyeball

conjunctivitis (pink eye) inflammation of the conjunctiva

cornea the clear, round, central window in the front of the eyeball overlying the pupil through which light travels to enter the eye

corneal abrasion a scratch on the cornea

corneal transplant a surgical procedure to replace a diseased cornea with a healthy donor cornea

corneal ulcer a deep infection in the cornea

cranial nerve one of twelve specialized nerves from the brain that control different parts of the eye, head, neck, and chest

cryotherapy freezing treatment

cystoid macular edema a disease in which fluid leaks into the macula and collects to form cysts

dacryocystitis infection of the tear drainage system

dacryocystorhinostomy (DCR) a surgical procedure to repair a blocked tear drainage system

diabetes mellitus a disease of abnormal blood sugar regulation

diabetic macular edema swelling in the central retina caused by diabetes

diabetic retinopathy a retinal disease caused by diabetes

dilation the process of enlarging the pupil with eye drops so that the back of the eye can be examined

diplopia double vision

dislocated lens a lens or lens implant that moves out of the capsular bag; or a lens or lens implant that moves out of the proper position along with the capsular bag

drusen aging deposits located under the retina

dry eye syndrome an abnormality of the tear film that lubricates the surface of the eye

dynamic wrinkles wrinkles that occur with facial expressions

ectropion an outward turning of the eyelid margin away from the eyeball

edema swelling

electroretinogram a special electrical test used mainly to examine retinal function

endophthalmitis a severe infection inside the eyeball

entropion an inward turning of the eyelid margin toward the eyeball

epiretinal membrane (cellophane retinopathy, macular pucker, preretinal gliosis) a thin sheet of abnormal scar tissue that grows over the retina

episclera the connective tissue layer between the conjunctiva and the sclera

episcleritis inflammation of the episclera

esotropia misalignment of an eye, in toward the nose

exotropia misalignment of an eye, out toward the ear on the same side

eye MD (ophthalmologist) a medical doctor trained to perform eye surgery who examines and treats all eye conditions

eye socket (orbit) the cavity in the head in which the eyeball sits

eyelid margin the edge of the eyelid where eyelashes grow

festoon a lower bag that forms between the lower eyelid and the cheek with aging

floater a spot that appears to drift in one's visual field, usually because of an opacity in the vitreous cavity

fluorescein angiogram a special photographic dye test used to examine the retina

focal laser a laser technique used mainly to treat macular edema

Fuchs endothelial corneal dystrophy a condition with abnormal corneal endothelial cells leading to corneal swelling and decreased vision

fundus autofluoresence is an imaging technique used to evaluate the health of the retina and the retinal pigment epithelium

fusion the ability of the brain to process and blend images coming from both eyes

giant cell arteritis (temporal arteritis) an inflammatory disease of blood vessels

glaucoma a disease of the optic nerve, often associated with high eye pressure

Graves' disease an autoimmune disorder that is the most common cause of hyperthyroidism

grid laser a laser technique used mainly to treat macular edema

hemoglobin A1c a blood test that measures the average blood sugar level over the previous three months

herniate to bulge or pouch forward

high-order aberrations optical imperfections that can distort the quality of vision and are not correctable by glasses or contact lenses

hordeolum (stye) a nodule of inflammation and infection that forms a bump in the eyelid

human immunodeficiency virus (HIV) the virus that causes Acquired Immune Deficiency Syndrome (AIDS)

hyperopia farsightedness

hypertension high blood pressure

hypertensive retinopathy a retinal disease caused by high blood pressure

hyperthyroidism overactivity of the thyroid gland

hypertropia misalignment of an eye upward

hyphema blood in the anterior chamber of the eye

hypotony low eye pressure

hypotropia misalignment of an eye downward

idiopathic intracranial hypertension (pseudotumor cerebri) a disease in which cerebrospinal fluid pressure is elevated without a known cause

indocyanine green angiography (ICGA) an imaging technique that uses a contrast dye to view the blood vessels behind the retina

intraocular foreign body an object inside the eyeball that is not naturally found there

iris the colored, circular part of the eye that surrounds the pupil

keratitis inflammation of the cornea

keratoconus a condition in which the cornea is abnormally steep and cone-shaped

laceration a wound or tear

lacrimal gland an orbital structure responsible for producing tears

LASEK (laser-assisted subepithelial keratectomy) a type of refractive surgery designed to improve one's unaided vision

laser retinopexy a laser technique used mainly to "tack down" the retina surrounding a retinal tear

laser skin resurfacing a technique in which a specialized laser is used to tighten the skin

laser trabeculoplasty a laser technique used mainly to treat certain types of glaucoma

LASIK (laser-assisted in situ keratomileusis) a type of refractive surgery designed to improve one's unaided vision

lens the lentil-shaped part of the eye behind the pupil that helps to focus light

leukocoria a white pupil limbus the outer edge of the cornea

lumbar puncture (spinal tap) a test in which a sample of the fluid that surrounds the spinal cord and brain is withdrawn and examined

macula the central area of the retina, responsible for central vision

macular edema swelling in the central retina

macular hole a hole in the central retina

macular ischemia reduced blood flow to the macula

macular pucker (cellophane retinopathy, epiretinal membrane, preretinal gliosis) a thin sheet of abnormal scar tissue that grows over the retina

macular translocation a rarely performed surgical technique to move the macula of the retina to a new location; used mainly for certain types of age-related macular degeneration

magnetic resonance imaging scan (MRI scan) a specialized imaging technique that uses a strong magnetic field and radio waves to visualize the organs and tissues inside the body

malignant cancerous

melanoma a cancer of pigment-containing cells in the skin or eye

meninges the three layers of tissue that surround the optic nerve and brain

metastatic a cancer that has spread from another part of the body

migraine an attack of neurologic or mood disturbance which often, but not always, includes headache

multiple sclerosis (MS) a disease of the brain and spinal cord in which the body attacks its own central nervous system

myopia nearsightedness

neovascular glaucoma glaucoma caused by growth of abnormal new blood vessels in the drain of the eye

neovascularization growth of abnormal new blood vessels

neuro-ophthalmologist an eye MD who specializes in the optic nerves and the eyes' connections to the brain

nevus a mole or pigmented lesion found on the skin or in the eye

occipital lobe the part of the brain located at the back of the head where vision is processed

ocular prosthesis an artificial eyeball that does not see

ocular ultrasound a procedure that uses sound waves to image ocular structures

ocularist a professional who specializes in making ocular prostheses

oculoplastic surgery a subspecialty field of ophthalmology that is concerned with cosmetic and functional aspects of the tissues surrounding the eyeballs

open globe a condition in which there is a full-thickness wound to the wall of the eyeball

ophthalmic allied health professional providers who make up the eye care team and include Certified Ophthalmic Assistants, Certified Ophthalmic Technicians, and Certified Ophthalmic Medical Technologists

ophthalmologist (eye MD) a medical doctor trained to perform eye surgery who examines and treats all eye conditions

opportunistic infection an infection that attacks weak, but not healthy, immune systems

optic canal a passageway through which nerves and blood vessels travel between the eye and the brain

optic chiasm an area in the brain where the optic nerves are joined

optic nerve the part of the eye that carries visual information from the eyeball to the brain

optic nerve sheath decompression a surgical procedure to relieve pressure on the optic nerve from its surrounding fluid

optic neuritis inflammation of the optic nerve

optic neuropathy abnormal function of the optic nerve

optic radiations nerve fibers in the brain that carry information from the optic tracts to the visual cortex

optic tract a structure in the brain that carries information from the optic chiasm to the optic radiations

optical coherence tomogram (OCT) a special non-contact, non-radiation, imaging technique that uses light waves to examine the optic nerve and retinal layers

optical coherence tomography angiography (OCT-A) a non-invasive imaging method that uses OCT technology to create a detailed three-dimensional map of the blood flow in the retina

optician an eye care professional who fits and dispenses corrective eyewear

optometrist an eye care professional who examines the eye, prescribes glasses and contact lenses, and medically treats certain eye conditions

ora serrata the part of the eyeball just behind the ciliary body where the retina ends

orbit (eye socket) the cavity in the head in which the eyeball sits

orbital blow-out fracture a break in one or more of the bones that make up the orbit and surround the eyeball

orbital cellulitis an infection in the orbit

orbital ecchymosis (black eye) a collection of fluid and blood in the tissues around the eye

orbital septum a thin layer of tissue behind the eyelids that helps prevent eyelid infections from reaching the orbit

pachymetry a technique used to measure the thickness of the cornea

panretinal laser photocoagulation (PRP) a laser technique used mainly to treat retinal neovascularization

papilledema swelling of the optic nerves caused by increased cerebrospinal fluid pressure around the brain

pars planitis inflammation in the front and middle parts of the eyeball

peripheral iridectomy a surgical or laser technique in which a tiny hole is made in the iris to prevent or treat certain types of glaucoma

phacoemulsification a method of surgically removing a cataract using ultrasound

photodynamic therapy (PDT) a special laser treatment used to treat certain types of wet age-related macular degeneration

photoreceptor a specialized cell in the retina that converts light images into electrical signals

pingueculum a benign growth that develops on the conjunctiva

pink eye (conjunctivitis) inflammation of the conjunctiva

pneumatic retinopexy a special technique involving cryotherapy and bubble injections to treat certain retinal detachments

polycarbonate an impact-resistant material used in the lenses of eyeglasses

posterior capsular opacity ("after cataract") a film that forms behind a lens implant

posterior chamber the space inside the eyeball between the back of the iris and the front of the vitreous gel

posterior vitreous detachment separation of the vitreous gel from the inner surface of the retina

preretinal gliosis (cellophane retinopathy, epiretinal membrane, macular pucker) a thin sheet of abnormal scar tissue that grows over the retina

presbyopia decreased ability to see near objects that occurs with aging

preseptal cellulitis infection of the eyelids and surrounding skin and soft tissues

PRK (photorefractive keratectomy) a type of refractive surgery designed to improve one's unaided vision

pseudotumor cerebri (idiopathic intracranial hypertension) a disease in which cerebrospinal fluid pressure is elevated without a known cause

pterygium (surfer's eye) a benign wedge-shaped growth over the conjunctiva that can extend onto the clear

ptosis a drooping upper eyelid

pupil the dark, round space in the center of the iris

radial keratotomy (RK) an early refractive surgery technique designed to improve one's unaided level of vision

red-green color deficiency an inherited difficulty in distinguishing between the colors red and green

refract to bend light

refraction testing a person's vision to determine the correct prescription for corrective lenses

refractive surgery a group of surgical techniques designed to improve one's unaided level of vision

retina a thin layer of complex nerve tissue that lines the inside back wall of the eyeball

retinal artery occlusion blockage of an artery that supplies blood to the retina

retinal break a hole or tear in the retina

retinal detachment an abnormal separation of the retina from the inner wall of the eyeball

retinal vein occlusion blockage of a vein that drains blood from the retina

retinitis pigmentosa a group of inherited retinal degenerative diseases

retinoblastoma a cancer of primitive retinal cells that grows inside the eyeball

rod a type of photoreceptor that processes dark and light images

sclera the white, outer layer of the eyeball

scleral buckling a surgical technique to treat retinal detachments

scleritis inflammation of the sclera

sebaceous cell carcinoma a rare cancer arising from eyelid oil glands

silicone oil a special material used to fill the eyeball after certain vitrectomy surgeries

slit lamp an illuminating microscope used to examine the front part of the eye

spinal tap (lumbar puncture) a test in which a sample of the fluid that surrounds the spinal cord and brain is withdrawn and examined

squamous cell carcinoma a type of skin cancer

static wrinkles wrinkles that are present when the face is still

stereopsis depth perception

steroid a type of anti-inflammatory medication

strabismus misalignment of one or both eyes

stroke a disease in which brain tissue is damaged by lack of blood supply

stye (hordeolum) a nodule of inflammation and infection that forms a bump in the eyelid

subconjunctival hemorrhage a collection of blood that accumulates under the conjunctiva

subluxed lens a lens or lens implant that shifts but stays within the capsular bag

surfer's eye (pterygium) a benign wedge-shaped growth over the conjunctiva that can extend onto the cornea

tarsorrhaphy a surgical procedure to attach the eyelids together

temporal arteritis (giant cell arteritis) an inflammatory disease of blood vessels

thyroid eye disease a set of eye problems typically associated with thyroid disease

toric a type of contact lens or lens implant that corrects astigmatism

trabeculectomy a type of glaucoma surgery

uveal tract the pigmented portion of the eyeball that includes the iris, ciliary body, and choroid

uveitis inflammation of the uveal tract inside the eyeball

verteporfin (Visudyne) a special dye used in photodynamic therapy

viral retinitis inflammation of the retina caused by a virus

virus an organism that lives by infecting other living cells

vision rehabilitation specialist a professional who helps people with impaired vision maximize their vision so that they can perform daily activities

visual acuity a person's level of vision

visual cortex the area of the brain at the back of the head where vision is processed

visual field entire space that can be seen without moving the eyes at a given time, includes both central and peripheral vision

Visudyne (verteporfin) a special dye used in photodynamic therapy

vitrectomy a surgical procedure to remove the vitreous from the vitreous cavity in the back of the eyeball

vitreous the natural gel that fills the back of the eyeball

vitreous cavity the space in the eyeball that contains the vitreous

wavefront a type of technology used to customize refractive surgery for each individual patient

x-linked an inheritance pattern in which mothers pass a gene to their children but only their sons usually show the effect of the gene

zonule a fiber that holds the capsular bag and lens in position

Contributors

Natalie A. Afshari, MD
Shiley Eye Institute, La Jolla, CA

Rosanna P. Bahadur, MD
Private practice, Jackson, MS

Paramjit K. Bhullar, MD
Duke Eye Center, Durham, NC

Faith A. Birnbaum, MD
Duke Eye Center, Durham, NC

Cassandra C. Brooks, MD
Duke Eye Center, Durham, NC

Pratap Challa, MD
Duke Eye Center, Durham, NC

Melissa Mei-Hsia Chan, MBBS
*Duke-National University of Singapore
Medical School, Singapore*

Ravi Chandrashekhar, MD, MSEE
Private practice, Dallas, TX

Nathan Cheung, OD, FAAO
Duke Eye Center, Durham, NC

Claudia S. Cohen, MD
Private practice, McLean, VA

Vincent A. Deramo, MD
Private practice, Long Island, NY

Cathy DiBernardo, RN
Duke Eye Center, Durham, NC

Laura B. Enyedi, MD
Duke Eye Center, Durham, NC

Sharon Fekrat, MD
Duke Eye Center, Durham, NC

Henry L. Feng, MD
Duke Eye Center, Durham, NC

Brenton D. Finklea, MD
Duke Eye Center, Durham, NC

Anna Ginter, MD
Duke Eye Center, Durham, NC

Tanya S. Glaser, MD
Duke Eye Center, Durham, NC

Michelle Sy Go, MS, MD
Duke Eye Center, Durham, NC

Mark Goerlitz-Jessen, MD
Duke Eye Center, Durham, NC

Herb Greenman, MD
Private practice, Charlotte, NC

Abhilash Guduru, MD
Duke Eye Center, Durham, NC

Preeya Gupta, MD
Duke Eye Center, Durham, NC

Renee Halberg, MSW, LCSW
Duke Eye Center, Durham, NC

S. Tammy Hsu, MD
Duke Eye Center, Durham, NC

Alessandro Iannaccone, MD, MS,
FARVO
Duke Eye Center, Durham, NC

Charlene L. James, OD
Duke Eye Center, Durham, NC

Kim Jiramongkolchai, MD
Wilmer Eye Institute,
Johns Hopkins, Baltimore, MD

Michael P. Kelly, FOPS
Duke Eye Center, Durham, NC

Muge R. Kesen, MD
Private practice, Gainesville, FL

Kirin Khan, MD
Duke Eye Center, Durham, NC

Wajiha Jurdi Kheir, MD
Duke Eye Center, Durham, NC

Jane S. Kim, MD
Duke Eye Center, Durham, NC

Jennifer Lira, MD
Private practice, Hickory, NC

Katy C. Liu, MD, PhD
Duke Eye Center, Durham, NC

Ramiro S. Maldonado, MD
University of Kentucky, Lexington

Ankur Mehra, MD
University of Kentucky, Lexington

Onyemaechi Nwanaji-Enwerem, MS
Duke University School of Medicine,
Durham, NC, and Harvard Kennedy
School

Priyatham S. Mettu, MD
Duke Eye Center, Durham, NC

Prithvi Mruthyunjaya, MD, MHS
Byers Eye Institute, Stanford,
Palo Alto, CA

Nisha Mukherjee, MD
Durham VA Medical Center,
Durham, NC

Kenneth Neufeld, MD
Private practice, Atlanta, GA

Kristen M. Peterson, MD
Private practice, Marietta, GA

James H. Powers, MD
Duke Eye Center, Durham, NC

S. Grace Prakalapakorn, MD, MPH
Duke Eye Center, Durham, NC

Michael S. Quist, MD
Duke Eye Center, Durham, NC

Leon Rafailov, MD
Duke Eye Center, Durham, NC

Roshni Ranjit-Reeves, MD
Duke Eye Center, Durham, NC

Nikolas Raufi, MD
Duke Eye Center, Durham, NC

William Raynor, BS
Duke Eye Center, Durham, NC

Cason Robbins, BS
Duke Eye Center, Durham, NC

Ananth Sastry, MD
Duke Eye Center, Durham, NC

Dianna L. Seldomridge, MD, MBA
Duke Eye Center, Winston-Salem, NC

Terry Semchyshyn, MD
Duke Eye Center, Winston-Salem, NC

Ann Shue, MD
Byers Eye Institute, Stanford,
Palo Alto, CA

Julia Song, MD
Private practice, Pasadena, CA

Brian Stagg, MD
Moran Eye Center, Salt Lake City, UT

Christopher Sun, MBBS
Duke-National University of Singapore
Medical School, Singapore

Anthony Therattil, BS
Duke Eye Center, Durham, NC

Daniel S. W. Ting, MD, PhD
Duke-National University of Singapore
Medical School, Singapore

Fay Jobe Tripp, MS, OTR/L,
CLVT, CDRS
Duke Eye Center, Durham, NC

Obinna Umunakwe, MD, PhD
Duke Eye Center, Durham, NC

Lejla Vajzovic, MD
Duke Eye Center, Durham, NC

Susan M. Wakil, MD
Duke Eye Center, Durham, NC

C. Ellis Wisely, MD, MBA
Duke Eye Center, Durham, NC

Julie A. Woodward, MD
Duke Eye Center, Durham, NC